LET'S TALK ABOUT DEATH

Breaking through old traditions and
looking for a new peaceful approach

M. Maurice Abitbol, M.D.

SPUYTEN DUYVIL

New York City

Abitbol, M. Maurice.
Let's talk about death : breaking through old traditions and looking for a new peaceful
approach / M. Maurice Abitbol.
p. ; cm.
Includes bibliographical references.
ISBN 978-1-933132-60-0
1. Terminal care. 2. Palliative treatment. 3. Terminally ill--Psychology. 4. Death. I.
Title.
[DNLM: 1. Attitude to Death. 2. Palliative Care. 3. Right to Die. 4. Terminal Care. 5.
Terminally Ill--psychology. BF 789.D4 A149L 2007]
R726.8.A233 2007
616'.029--dc22
2007036953

TABLE OF CONTENTS

Chapter 1

THE REVOLUTIONARY CONCEPT OF A BETTER DEATH

One has to die sometime...

Considering how much we've improved every aspect of our lives, it's a mystery why we haven't learned how to die better deaths. From the very beginning, we have known nothing but cruel, brutal or painful death. We have been conditioned to expect death and dying to be completely negative experiences; anything else is inconceivable.

Death is the one area that has resisted our innate and often ingenious impulse to improve the human condition. We have improved our method of birth through prenatal and obstetrical care, our growth into adulthood through pediatric care, the quality of our entire adult life through health and social advances, and even our old age through everything from exercise and diet to Social Security and Medicare.

The first sustained criticisms of our way of death emerged in the '60s, but they focused on a tangential issue. "The High Cost of Dying" (Economist, 9/16/62) and "Can You Afford to Die?" (The Saturday Evening Post, 6/17/61), were two early articles that made people aware of how costly funerals have become. Financial shenanigans, however, hurt only our pocketbooks. The real harm is the tremendous emotional and social turmoil that results from the way we approach death and how we deal with people in the terminal stage of life.

Historically, death always has been a horror to mankind. What scares me, and what I will illustrate in this book, is that we're making it worse. Our current treatment exacerbates the fear of death and interferes with our ability to lead a normal, happy life; we are exposed to death constantly, not just when we're dying. As witnesses to the deaths of others and given the horrible ways they die, our fear of death begins early and builds as we age.

Life has the potential to be a beautiful, enjoyable and even ecstatic experience, but we sometimes fail to realize this potential because of our ignorance, hostility, sadism and masochism. I take no pride in adding another item to this list. Increasingly, life is much less than it could be because of our approach to death and dying. We unnecessarily diminish the quality of our lives, especially in old age. We possess the capabilities to face death calmly and peacefully, but we don't use them. The fact that we don't is a crime, and it is what compels me to take a stance that I'm sure will offend some of my medical brethren and others in the healthcare community.

In the following pages, I will describe how the circumstances surrounding death can be improved. I will demonstrate that our current fear of death is out of proportion to the reality of death. If we scale down the concept of death and approach it more rationally and less hysterically, it can be dealt with in a way that enhances our quality of life.

On the Battle Lines: The Making of a Revolutionary

My interest in the study of death and dying started early in my medical career when I disciplined myself to be simultaneously subjective and objective. I learned to be objective in order to apply the science of medicine and subjective to apply the art. In other words, I tried to be open-minded and holistic when pure science didn't work or when another, better option might exist. Taking my cue from Descartes, I became curious and doubted many accepted practices and principles, especially when it came to dying and death. I re-evaluated every aspect concerning the medical and social approaches to dealing with dying patients. By opening myself to the feelings of terminally ill patients and attempting to understand their state of mind, I gradually acquired an unusual expertise outside my area of specialization. Though this expertise may have given rise to revolutionary ideas about death, it's also helped me translate them into very practical suggestions and concepts that would be relatively easy to implement.

I've spent a good portion of my free time reflecting on the cases of dying patients I've treated. I've also investigated death and dying throughout history and in various cultures. I've talked with physicians, psychologists, psychiatrists, religious ministers, philosophers, and various scientists about the problems that arise when we confront death.

Much of my work in this area hits close to home. As a doctor, I've been told by all types of patients that they find medicine and the ways of physicians and hospitals to be cloaked in mystery. This mystery deepens when it comes to the management of dying patients. Fear, guilt, denial, and fantasy predominate when someone is dying because even though we're all obsessed with death, we avoid talking about it. This obsessive silence has led to the belief that the real death process is carried out only by doctors in emergency rooms and hospitals. This is a logical (if erroneous) conclusion since most dying patients are rushed to emergency rooms and hospitals in the hope of preventing death. We leave emergency rooms and hospitals with the unarticulated conviction that somewhere within those walls resides the mysterious mechanism for making death. It's assumed that doctors hold the key to unlocking this mystery. This misconception is reinforced by the many types of gadgets attached to dying patients. The average person has little understanding about what all the highly sophisticated technology does, and in lieu of this understanding, he assumes that this is the only possible place where the process of death can unfold.

Today, death rarely occurs at home with each member of the family witnessing the progressive decline of life and approach of death while the religious minister and close friends are comforting the dying patient. Death is now a secret event with all kinds of medical professionals hovering around the dying patient speaking an arcane language. Anyone who has observed this process knows that there's a ritualistic quality to it; it verges on being a secret ceremony. Most people are afraid to miss this ceremony; they don't dare die in any place other than a hospital or emergency room surrounded by the high priests of medicine. Even in an age of malpractice suits, doctors retain a shamanistic quality, and perhaps people feel they need to die with doctors close by.

Most physicians argue that it is the role of the medical profession to fight death at all costs. When death becomes inevitable as a result of widespread cancer or the failure of a vital organ, however, perhaps the medical treatment of the terminally ill patient should end right there.

At a certain point after I had seen one too many patients die horrible deaths, I began to wonder if a completely different approach should be considered. Even early in my career, I struggled with how to deal differently with dying patients. If I were dispassionate, I could keep a clear mind and better manage the cases. If I were to express my emotions, I could empathize with patients and let them know I cared. It soon dawned on me that neither approach was effective. It also became clear that the medical profession wasn't particularly concerned about exploring in any depth the treatment issues related to dying patients. I wondered if they were right; if doctors weren't the right people to deal with terminally ill patients?

Yet if you think about it, who is in a better position to deal with individuals who are dying? Doctors are the only ones who can prescribe the drugs patients require; they are the ones who are most familiar with the course a given disease will take and can prepare people accordingly; they're the ones who have the knowledge to guide patients through the choices that present themselves in the final months, weeks and days of their lives.

Given this responsibility, what should we do with it? Given that our current approach is abysmal, what other options are there? Any student of history and of different cultures knows that different approaches exist. Our man-made rules need to be questioned, and the environment is becoming increasingly receptive to this questioning. To start this process, we must investigate all the factors that contribute to our current approach and discover why certain feelings and fears are activated when death approaches. This book is part of that investigation.

Fighting Versus Acceptance

I don't want to make it sound like it will be easy to change our approach to death and dying. Changing any cultural norm is difficult. We're up against a belief that has survived for many generations and been integrated into the healthcare culture. It's a belief that doctors, hospital administrators and other healthcare professionals have vigorously maintained. In a nutshell, that belief is as follows:

We will reject death and extend life for as long as possible.

On the surface, such a belief sounds noble and serves as a mantra for idealistic doctors. There is an almost religious fervor to the way in which we worship an extended life and view death as the devil's work. The temples are hospitals, emergency rooms and offices of medical specialists. The religious ministers are the doctors. The organizers of this cult are the health system, lawyers, and indirectly the politicians and news media, who want to burn the heretics—they ostracize anyone who dares suggest that the plug be pulled, that euthanasia is a viable option. All this made me question the medical profession's role of providing care to a terminally ill patient. Why did physicians end up with such an awesome responsibility, since we have no training for it and very often lack the emotional strength and maturity to deal with this condition. This is the first time in history that the medical profession has assumed a mortuary function, and even now it's the norm only in Western cultures.

Based on my experiences and research, I don't believe that our current mode of death is natural. While we die natural biological deaths, they are unnatural from a human point of view. For most people, death comes as an unexpected and usually dreaded catastrophe. Psychologically and emotionally, we reject death as traumatic, cruel, and inhumane. We can rationalize all we want that "one has to die sometime", but we don't have to die in such an unnaturally fearful, traumatized state.

Given our fear, our approach to death is and always has been disorganized. The isolated individual has never been able to prepare for his own death, and when death eventually comes, systems, customs, traditions, religious beliefs and individual or mass hysteria have taken over the dying process. On a medical level, management of dying patients involves approaches that are contradictory, haphazard, sometimes useless and harmful and always very costly. As a result of all this, the individual has little control over how he dies.

It has reached a point where talking about death is almost a taboo in our culture. The terminally ill patient, as well as his friends, family, doctors and nurses, have nothing else on their minds except how to ignore and delay death for as long as possible. Today, a hero is no longer one who faces inevitable death with courage and serenity, but one who fights it to the bitter end. The poet Dylan Thomas advised, Do not go gentle into that good night/rage, rage against the close of day. It's good poetry but bad policy; we need to learn to make peace with the fact of our own mortality.

We do not know how to become old and die, and this is a modern tragedy. I believe that our changing condition of life requires a changing approach to death, and we have not yet made the transition. We're incapable of dealing with death in a sane and sensitive way.

It's time for us to exert more control over how we die, and I hope this book provides the inspiration and ideas for doing so. The great irony is that though we constantly choose our life, we rarely choose our death. We simply submit to what fate and healthcare professionals hand us. Why not take advantage of scientific progress to devise a more satisfactory end? In the following pages, you'll find a number of feasible suggestions in this regard.

Whether or not we want to admit it, death is the most significant aspect of our life. On the surface, we may ignore or block it completely, refuse to discuss it and even panic when we think about it. Yet it's always there, roiling about in the back of our minds. We are preoccupied with death, and the precautions we take to stay alive are boundless. It would not be too far off base to define life as the avoidance of death.

That's a sad definition. We don't have to live our life in constant fear, and one of my goals in writing this book is to relieve the terrible anxiety and dread that dominates our waking lives and our dreams. By understanding and analyzing what death is, our feelings about it and alternative ways of dying, we can make great strides in lessening our anxiety.

Our obsession with death has produced many books on this subject. The Tibetan Book of the Dead by Evans-Wentz (1960) makes us aware of the Eastern concept of death as opposed to the Western concept. On Death and Dying by Kübler-Ross (1970) is certainly a major teaching source and considered a classic by many. Embraced by the Light by Eadie (1992), Transformed by the Light by Morse (1992), and Seattle International Association of Near Death Studies all have described the mystic experience of near-death. How We Die: Reflections on Life's Final Chapter by Nuland (1994) illuminates the physiology of death. The Space of Death by Ragon (1983) studies the archeology of death.

As many and varied as these books are, none of them proposes a revolutionary change in the way in which we approach and manage dying. This is a manifesto of sorts, but a practical one. I don't intend to deal only in theory and abstract concepts, but to offer implementable ideas and resources based on real life-and-death stories.

In my investigations, I've discovered many compelling stories and ideas. Some of them, however, are not always easy to take. It requires a certain amount of courage to read the heartbreaking stories of people who died in pain and fear. It demands a degree of fortitude to contemplate many of the issues I will raise. Even though you don't know the people discussed in this book and will probably live for many more years, every death touches us. In a strange but vivid way, we experience death in a limited dimension each time someone dies. Not only is there concern and empathy for others, but we ourselves are also witness to and involved with another's death—it reminds us that sooner or later, that person will be us.

As scary as that thought might be, my purpose is not to scare you but help you come to terms with that fear. The good news is that all of us have the ability to handle it, and that we possess the technology, the medicine and the strength and wisdom of the human race to handle it effectively.

Chapter 2

GOOD AND BAD DEATHS:
WHAT WE CAN LEARN FROM OTHER PEOPLE'S STORIES

I believe it's important for you to understand the experiences that have shaped my perspective on death. I'd like to share some case histories with you, both from my medical and my personal life. More than anything else I could write, these stories illustrate what's wrong with our way of death and why dying fills us with dread. A few of them, however, provide hope for an alternative.

As pessimistic as some of the stories are, I am optimistic that we can change how we deal with death. We can improve the quality of death the same way we have improved the quality of life. I am convinced that our culture possesses all the necessary tools to create a peaceful and harmonious death.

The problem, of course, is that the concept of dreadful death has a tremendous hold on us. We're acutely aware of the disorganized interference that takes place when someone is dying, and this specter hovers over us and comes to haunt us when it's our time. Yet this fear is so much a part of our culture, we consider it natural and normal.

Much of our fear can be traced to medical and hospital practices and our misunderstanding of them. With all the recent advances in the medical field, especially as they apply to terminal conditions, there is more complexity and confusion than ever before. By revealing why healthcare professionals do the things they do, I hope to demystify the process. The greatest fear is that of the unknown, and I trust that by making certain practices and procedures known, I can reduce the level of fear. The stories in this chapter will at least start the process of demystification.

I have practiced obstetrics and gynecology for forty years specializing in malignancies of the female genital organs. During my career, I have had ample opportunities to observe and treat dying patients as well as witness the reaction of their families. I have closely followed more than one hundred dying patients, and I have selected the majority of stories in this chapter from that group.

Many patients I discuss here died of cancer, so I believe it would be helpful if I gave you a quick overview of the disease. Cancer is a mysterious and maybe an inevitable process of healthy cells becoming malignant. As our life expectancy increases, we are more likely to get cancer. We do not know why a cell becomes cancerous, no more than we know why a cell lives or eventually dies. A normal living cell grows and multiplies in an orderly and determined manner, allowing the cells and the tissues or organs formed by these cells to fulfill their functions in the body. It is not well understood how the growth and multiplication of the body cells are normally controlled. We do know that this cell growth and multiplication may spiral out of control. Growth and multiplication then becomes rapid, disorganized, and a tumor or growth is formed. It is hypothesized that a *single* cell has escaped control and that is all it takes to start a tumor. The malignant tumors become invasive and destructive by spreading to all surrounding organs (for instance, cancer of the cervix will extend to the vagina, bladder, rectum). They also metastasize, meaning that the malignant cells are transplanted to distant locations where they keep multiplying and interfere with other organs of the body. Eventually, interference with one or several organs leads to death. Even if no vital organ is seriously interfered with, however, the whole body is malignantly poisoned, resulting in a slow deterioration and emaciation that ends in death.

The present treatment of malignancies is rather simple and has changed little during this century although these modes of treatment continuously have been improved. There are and have been only three basic modes of treatment (which are used singly or in combination):

Surgery. The tumor is cut out. The hope is to remove not only the tumor itself but also its surrounding tissue. This surgery is rather delicate to perform and highly specialized because it involves separating the malignant from the healthy tissues and involves removal of the regional lymph nodes (very often a procedure of doubtful value).

There is really no surgical treatment for metastases because when a metastasis is recognized in one organ, it is generally assumed that there are metastases in other organs.

Radiotherapy. The tumor and its surrounding tissue are burned. Malignant cells are more sensitive to radiation than non-malignant cells. By careful radiation dosage skillfully directed to the tumor site, one can hope to destroy the tumor tissue with minimal damage to the healthy tissue. Usually radiation is reserved for a tumor that has spread beyond surgical removal or tumors that are located in sites that pose difficult or dangerous access. It is also reserved for those patients whose general condition make them poor candidates for surgery.

Chemotherapy. The tumor cells are poisoned. The poison dose for the malignant cells is much lower than the poison dose for healthy tissue. By careful dosage planning, one can hope to regress, delay, or in some rare cases, cure a widespread malignancy. Chemotherapy is reserved for systemic malignancies (hematological or lymphatic system malignancies) or those malignancies that have widely metastasized.

Progress in treating cancer has been made in many fields. The most important and promising step is earlier recognition of the malignant tumor, not only in the early stages of malignancy, but also in the premalignant stages. Cancer of the uterus, uterine cervix, breast, colon, and prostate have been reduced. People have benefited from early diagnosis. The earlier the treatment, the better the chance for cure, and if the tumor is recognized at the premalignant stages, the chances of cure are almost total. Early diagnosis allows for early treatment that can more readily cure the tumor. Unfortunately, early malignancies or premalignant tumors have no overt signs or symptoms; the only solution is widespread education for the earliest signs and symptoms and frequent check-ups.

Other progress is recognition of causative or predisposing factors to malignancies. We know, for instance, that good sexual hygiene will diminish chances of cancer of the uterine cervix or penis. On the other hand, smoking predisposes to cancer of the lung. Most known predisposing factors are hypothetical however, usually unproved, and more often reported in the general magazines rather than in the scientific literature.

Understanding the basic causes of cancer has progressed more in theory than in practical applications. Scientific literature on this subject is immense. It is mostly composed of isolated observations on the biological and biochemical mechanisms of the process of malignancy. It frequently consists of hopes (that often prove false) associated with the promise of a cure within the next ten years. Today we know no more about the cause of cancer than we did at the beginning of the previous century. More than one century of continuous research in the cause and prevention of cancer has produced no breakthroughs. The treatment is still to surgically cut, burn by radiation, and poison with drugs, although these three modes of treatment continue to be improved.

Chemotherapy is an excellent tool that works very well in selected cases. It produces a noticeable remission and even cures in the early stages of lymphomas. It produces remarkable remission in some types of ovarian carcinoma. Just as often, however, it has no effect on the majority of widespread malignancies and the tumor keeps progressing up to the terminal stage. Chemotherapy is not a benign treatment. The average length of treatment is six months and sometimes longer. Its traumatic effects include loss of hair (temporarily), loss of appetite, sleeplessness and irritability and other unpleasant (and sometime debilitating) side-effects. All patients have undergone biopsies of their tumors, so that the nature and grading of the tumor are well known, and, with few exceptions, the response and non-response to chemotherapy is also known in advance. Therefore, an important percentage of patients with widespread cancer could be spared the unnecessary chemotherapy.

The scientific rationale for imposing chemotherapy on everyone is the rare but miraculous permanent cure of someone suffering from a widespread malignancy. I have no way of analyzing each and every miracle cure, but my experience with these so-called cures reveals that either there was a misdiagnosis or the malignancy was growing so slowly that any treatment (including no treatment) would have been effective.

All this provides you with a fitting preamble to the cases I'm about to share. I want you to understand not only the nature of the disease but my bias against unnecessary or harmful treatments and the false hope of a cure that it engenders.

Case 1: Miss Smith

Miss Smith was fifty years old, single, and a bookkeeper before her illness. She had ovarian cancer which had spread throughout her body. She was suffering from progressive intestinal obstruction, vomiting, and eventually became unable to eat. She was hospitalized for two weeks as her condition progressively deteriorated, and her only treatments were fluids given intravenously and sedation. As her condition worsened, she became emaciated and was unconscious for three or four days prior to her death. The nature of her condition was never discussed with her. She never asked. She had a brother from California who came to visit her once in the hospital, and a married sister whom she lived with and who visited her daily. Some colleagues from work dropped in occasionally during visiting hours and brought flowers and cards, and all said they hoped to see her back at work soon. She was Irish Catholic, and the priest visited her once the first day of her hospitalization, but she never asked to see him again.

Miss Smith was transferred to a room at the end of the corridor and visits by family, doctors, and nurses were always short. At the end of medical or nursing rounds, she was always asked, "Anything I can do for you?" and the answer always was "No, thank you." Sometimes the doctor would ask, "Do you have any questions?" or "Do you have any questions about your medical condition?" The answer always was the same, "No, thank you." She was not talkative, but as her condition worsened, she became increasingly

withdrawn, and almost never talked except when asked a question and her answers were always monosyllabic. It was not long before she died.

What We Can Learn From Miss Smith's Death

This case is typical of death today. Death is a blank, the subject skirted by the patient, friends, family and medical staff. Everyone behaves as if it does not exist, as if it is not going to happen. Miss Smith could have been being treated for a broken arm; no one prepared her for her death or allowed her to talk about it at length. Even the Catholic priest routinely visited her as he would any Catholic patient in the hospital. While the doctors and nurses discussed her worsening condition among themselves, they did not include Miss Smith in the discussion. Doctors told Miss Smith's family that she was going to die but never discussed the subject with them again after that first prognosis. According to medical, religious, social and legal standards, this is currently considered successful management of a dying patient.

It's considered successful management because healthcare professionals don't want to panic their patients. Everyone asks with great concern: Does the patient know she is dying? To make sure she does not know, people are very careful not to talk about this subject to the patient or within her hearing. The medical profession always has attempted to hide the deadly prognosis associated with malignancies by substituting complicated words. In Europe, doctors use the word neo (as in neoplasms) to imply malignant. Here the new phrase is mitotic figure implying proliferation of malignant cells. Family and friends carefully watch their language, avoiding discussion of death and always reassure the patient that she looks better and will soon recover.

If, at this stage of incurable disease and oncoming death, the family, doctors, or nurses are asked, "Why don't you want the patient to know that she is dying," invariably the answers include such concerns as: "She couldn't take it," "She could have a bad reaction," "She may become hysterical," or "She may jump out the window."

Perhaps the most sadistic element of this approach is that the patient is forced to cooperate in the charade. Even though most patients like Miss Smith know they're dying, they pretend they're not; they feel this denial is expected of them. They've learned to pretend because they've played this game with others. When Miss Smith was healthy, she too had told dying friends how well they looked and cheered them up by making plans for outings that would never happen. She knew the rules of how to talk to a dying patient, and she knew the rules of how a dying patient should respond.

Case 2: Mrs. Jones

Mrs. Jones, 50, was admitted to the hospital for vague generalized pain. During the previous year she had been operated on for cancer of the thyroid, and now the diagnostic workup showed widespread metastasis. Although she appeared to be in good health, it was obvious from the medical workup that she had only a few weeks to a couple of

months to live. When making my evening rounds I was prepared to give her the "You are doing fine" routine. She interrupted me suddenly and a bit angrily and told me of a long conversation she had had with her private physician that morning in which she had asked him for a complete and accurate report. He had told Mrs. Jones that her cancer was now generalized (she knew that her operation the previous year was for a malignancy), that she didn't have long to live, and prescribed various medications for her (which I will describe later). There was no panic on her part. She said she had led a full life, her children were almost grown, and her husband would recover.

What I vividly remember is my own state of panic in contrast to her relative calm. As long as I felt that I was in control of her process of dying, I was comfortable treating her condition in the traditional way. As soon as she took control, however, I was at a loss. Like many doctors (and other people, for that matter), I had become a slave of my routine.

What We Can Learn from Mrs. Jones' Death

Mrs. Jones helped me understand that I was wrong to impose my way of facing death on patients. The dying patient should be allowed to approach death her own way, and the outsider's role should be to support, assist, and even direct the dying patient to take whatever path toward death she wishes.

I also came to the rather startling conclusion that the dying person is not the only one who is weak and desperate; that doctors are just as likely to experience these feelings. The difference is that doctors can safely repress their fear of death and concentrate on the dying person's fear. The dying person, on the other hand, may be consciously fearful of death but imagines that doctors don't harbor similar feelings.

Third, after treating Mrs. Jones, I determined that the worst aspect of the dying process is isolation. The anxiety and fear of dying isolates the patient. No one is available to communicate all the thoughts roiling in her mind. Mrs. Jones was able to shatter that isolation because she was aware of exactly what her condition entailed and could share her feelings with her private physician, with me as the resident making rounds and with her husband and children. No one tiptoed around the fact of her dying; everyone accepted it and allowed her to talk about it. Her private physician told me later that as her pain and discomfort increased, she received higher doses of morphine orally, then continuously through an intravenous line. She died peacefully in the arms of her husband, who each year sends a card to the private physician thanking him for the way he treated his wife.

Case 3: Mrs. Rivers

This forty-six-year-old woman was dying of uterine cervix cancer that had spread to other organs (bladder, rectum, lymph nodes, etc.). Mrs. Rivers had a strong will to live; she was responsible for running a major business and took this responsibility seriously. Over the previous two years she had had several admissions to the hospital, and each time she had had an operation that diverted the function of a system blocked by the spreading malignancy. Mrs. Rivers required extensive treatment during her admissions, involving a range of doctors, nurses, personnel in the operating room and laboratories and others. No one told her she might die of the disease, and each operation she underwent was presented to her as a temporary inconvenience. The implicit and explicit message communicated was: Life would return to normal after the operation. On my daily rounds I helped deliver this message, and I was convinced she believed me. When Mrs. Rivers was admitted for yet another treatment, she died suddenly after all her body systems ceased to function.

A few days after her death, I received a letter from the priest who had visited her daily during her last hospital admission. He wrote that Mrs. Rivers had known for the last two years about her terminal condition and appreciated all the efforts we made to lengthen her life. With each admission, she had felt like asking us to stop our efforts but feared it would hurt the doctors' feelings. She apologized for all the useless effort her condition had required.

What We Can Learn from Mrs. Rivers' Death

The biggest mistake we made was not considering our surgical treatment from a whole patient perspective. The irony of the situation was that we were doing what we thought the patient wanted and the patient was going along quietly because she thought the surgery was what we wanted. If we had communicated better—if we had communicated in any meaningful way—we would have probably chosen a different and more humane course of action.

The last two years of Mrs. Rivers' life was unnecessarily chaotic and traumatic. At the very least, she certainly would have preferred to spend more time at home and less time in the hospital. It's instructive that she was able to talk about these issues with her priest but not with me or any other member of the hospital medical staff. As disheartening as this situation is, it also suggests that perhaps doctors need to become more willing to listen and less eager to rush to judgment.

Case 4: Mrs. Huskins

This middle-aged woman had a carcinoma of the ovary which had been operated on two years ago and was hospitalized because her malignancy had recurred and extended to every organ in her abdomen. First, Mrs. Huskins' colon was blocked, and she underwent a colostomy (an opening in her abdominal wall connected with a hole in her large bowel for evacuation of her feces). Then she had a nephrostomy (two holes in her back to evacuate her urine because her kidneys were blocked). After that she had a tracheostomy (a hole in her throat so she could breathe). During that time she was being artificially fed with intravenous fluids because she could not swallow. Finally, she went into cardiac arrest, had her chest opened for cardiac massage from which she never recovered, and she died. All these procedures were done with the patient's consent when she was conscious, or with her family's consent when she was not. Proudly, the physicians in charge bragged that they added one month to her life. Since the family was of average means and Mrs. Huskins lacked medical insurance, all of their savings were wiped out during this month of hospitalization. From what she said and the way she looked, Mrs. Huskins was clearly angry about everything she was going through and just wished to die.

What We Can Learn from Mrs. Huskins' Death

The hospital is not always the best place to die. When I suggested to Mrs. Huskins that she might be more comfortable at home, her family objected; one member of the family screamed, What will I do if she dies there? The family was as scared of Mrs. Hoskins' impending death as Mrs. Hoskins was. Many families are relieved when hospitals take care of the messy business of dying, and they don't have to deal with it directly. Certainly Mrs. Hoskins would have preferred to die at home. I'm sure she would have gladly sacrificed the additional month of life the doctors bragged about in exchange for a comfortable, familiar, pain-free environment.

Case 5: Ericka

Ericka was the wife of a close friend. She had widespread cancer that did not respond to multiple operations or repeated chemotherapy.

All she needed was intravenous fluids to extend her life a few weeks and sedation to relieve her increasing abdominal discomfort. Following my suggestion, she was taken home to die in the midst of her family.

I knew Ericka well, and I perceived that she desperately wanted to die at home away from the medical and nursing care in the hospital which she found aggravating. She wanted to be away from curious visitors who never respected the "do not disturb" sign on the door of her hospital room. She wanted to be with her family because, as she told me one day, "I am very concerned about how my husband and children will be affected after I am gone."

Unfortunately, conditions at home weren't much of an improvement. Her husband was deeply attached to Ericka and could not accept that she was going to die. She wanted to discuss her coming death with her husband and children, but her husband never allowed it. The children were never told the whole truth about their mother's approaching death until a few weeks before she died. One child reacted badly to the shock of this news, had a fight with his father and left home.

Ericka tried to communicate with her family about her coming death, and to tell them she was not afraid of dying. She wanted to say she was not frightened but did not want to scare anyone. This paradox made it difficult for her to articulate her feelings and ultimately she felt she couldn't communicate them to anyone in her family.

What We Can Learn From Ericka's Death

As much as I wish the solution were to have people die at home, it's not that simple. Though people certainly have more privacy at home and are free from a hospital's invasive procedures, they can be just as frightened and lonely at home as in a hospital. Despite being surrounded by her family, Ericka was isolated by her inability to communicate her feelings...and the inability of family members to help her do so.

Case 6: Julia

Julia's widespread cervical cancer had not responded to any treatment and eventually blocked the kidneys. When she asked me how long she had to live, I answered that it would be approximately two to three months. She asked if she was going to suffer, and I answered that I would take care of her while she was dying the way I took care of her while she was living. In other words, I would be honest with her, ease her pain and not subject her to unnecessary treatments. The reaction of the doctors, medical students, and nurses who witnessed the conversation was one of horror, and I was reported to the chief of the department for my cruelty. Nobody, however, paid any attention to the immediate reaction of the patient following this conversation. Julia applied make-up to her face with a generous amount of lipstick, walked out of the examination room with a peaceful smile and kissed her husband. Obviously, I had told her nothing she did not already suspect, and Julia's husband had asked me to give her this information. Julia did not want to leave an image of sadness, panic, or agony for her family and was ready to face death in a positive way.

I could have made two holes in her back for her to evacuate urine; I could have made a hole in her stomach for her to be fed artificially; I could have used a new experimental drug. All this may have given her a few more weeks of life under agonizing and costly conditions. She did not want that. Instead, I prescribed a generous amount of drugs to relieve her pain, tension, and anxiety. She preferred to stay in the hospital and her private room was transformed into a sort of family room where anyone she wished to see was free to come and go. One morning she was dead, but the evening before she was having a peaceful and joyous conversation with all her family around. Two years later I met her husband, who told me I had helped him through the most difficult part of his life without pain, anxiety, or guilt.

What We Can Learn From Julia's Death

For most of us, it's not as important where we die but how. I'm not sure if it's fair to call any death a good one, but Julia left this world with a sense of resolution and acceptance. I think we can all take hope from the fact that not only Julia but her husband found her death to be a natural ending to her life. It's possible to die with dignity and on your own terms.

Case 7: Eddy

I'd like to describe Eddy's death in more detail than the others because he died in a manner that approached ideal—or at least my ideal. When he was diagnosed with colon cancer, Eddy's disease was at an advanced stage and he was given about a year to live. Eddy was both a close friend and a doctor, and he shared a great deal with me during that final year.

Astute, intelligent and a great diagnostician, Eddy had blood in his stools for three years yet ignored the obvious warning signs. It seems likely that Eddy was in denial; how else to explain why he failed to undergo a complete diagnostic exam that could have saved his life and that he certainly would have ordered for any patient exhibiting this symptom?

Eddy was in his sixties, his children were grown, and he was not leaving any problems behind. He and I knew that when cancer spreads to the liver, a progressive coma results and the patient dies of liver insufficiency. Death from cancer of the liver, called hepatic coma, is a relatively painless way of dying, although it may last for a few weeks. When a patient has an incurable cancer, hepatic coma is always the preferred mode of death. On numerous occasions, Eddy and I had discussed the best way of dying, and how each of us would like his death to be. Like everyone else, we had always thought that the best way to die would be to go to sleep peacefully some evening and not wake up, as had happened once to a colleague of ours. Eddy's other stipulations about dying were: he did not want to die in pain; he did not want to finish his life as a cripple; and he did not want any stoma or artificial opening in his body.

Given his condition, I assumed that Eddy was going to be able to die as he wished. Nonetheless, I was nervous about broaching this subject with him, uncertain how he'd react. I will never forget our first meeting after the diagnosis of his extended cancer was established. Eddy informed me of the nature and extent of his disease, and immediately all the ironies and paradoxes of this situation came into play. On the one hand, I was concerned that his inevitable death was going to terrify him. On the other hand, he was concerned that his inevitable death was going to scare me since he knew very well that the living are, consciously or not, afraid of dying people. After we started to talk, however, it became clear that he was not afraid of dying and that realization helped me accept the fact of his dying without overwhelming fear.

Word of his condition spread among his friends and acquaintances, and expressions of false sympathy and fear created a vacuum around him. People either behaved normally (as if nothing were wrong) and insisted that he looked fine or they simply avoided him. These behaviors isolated Eddy, and I tried to avoid contributing to his isolation. I allowed him to talk about any subject including his death, and although he scared me sometimes, we met frequently. When he spoke about his concerns and fear about his death, I also mentioned my concerns and fear about his dying. I felt my presence was meaningful to him because it lessened his isolation.

Eddy became ecstatic upon learning his diagnosis. For some people, work loses all meaning once they know they're going to die. For Eddy—who had many patients—work became even more exciting and challenging, and he went about his job with renewed vigor. As Eddy said: "The experience of dying makes my life more meaningful, more complete...It looks like so far only one part of my brain was functioning, but now all the synapses of my brain have opened up. My whole brain is now fully functional. I feel like I am going through an ecstatic, cosmic experience."

Eddy's ecstasy manifested itself in various ways. He confided to me that the night after he learned about his widespread cancer, he had the most beautiful dream of his life. He dreamed that he was in heaven in different forms, with all kinds of friends and involved in all kinds of dynamic activities. The strange and fantastic aspect of this paradisiacal feeling is that it persisted after he woke.

He never interrupted his work as long as he had enough strength to do it, and his dynamism and happiness in doing it never diminished.

Although his office and hospital staff took great care to avoid bringing up Eddy's condition, he kept relating to everyone as usual.

Once the nature of the disease was known and the spread of the cancer determined, Eddy became very inquisitive about any procedure done to him. To perform a procedure to extend his life did not interest him at all; the prospect of a colostomy repulsed him. Chemotherapy interested him a little and he went along with it only because it did not produce any side-effect. All he wanted was to work as long as he could, obtain the proper medication for any discomfort or pain and stay at home with his family for as long as possible.

He wanted to determine as accurately as possible how his life would end. He insisted that he did not want to be bedridden and did not want any kind of artificial life support to prolong his ordeal. He did not want any resuscitation procedure and signed a DNR (do not resuscitate) order. He did not want to be a nuisance to himself or others.

Eddy was able to manage the process of dying to his satisfaction from start to finish. At the end, he went into a progressive coma, and I made sure that a continuous drip of intravenous morphine was running for his abdominal cramps.

Looking back, I recall a few times when Eddy became overwhelmed by his situation. He sometimes despaired at the thought of being gone while all those people he cared about remained alive. But these moments were brief and his predominant mood was euphoric. When the semi-coma began, with frequent episodes of full consciousness, he always mentioned the wonderful dreams he'd been having and other positive aspects of his life.

His family courageously fought against their own sadness. They recognized that this was how he wanted to die, and they were happy to do it his way; it would have been cruel on their part to spoil it by being upset and depressed. Eddy stressed that it made him feel good when everyone around him felt happy. He wanted them to share his calm and happiness. When a woman came to visit him one day and began to cry, he remonstrated with her by saying, "Let us not start that again; you hurt me that way."

Though Eddy's visitors always remarked on how good he looked and how well he seemed to be doing, none of them described his own emotional reaction to seeing him dying. None ever mentioned his personal terror at seeing Eddy dying. No one expressed his fear of death, anger, or confusion at seeing him dying so calmly and happily. A few of Eddy's close friends told me that the reason they did not visit him was because they did not know how to react; they were embarrassed and even afraid. One of his friends told me that he did not like to visit Eddy because he found him too calm.

What We Can Learn from Eddy's Death

Eddy was living his death process intensely and without fear. It made me wonder if there is something positive in the dying process that the average person is missing. Was I witnessing something unusual, almost unique, in Eddy's case, or was I witnessing something that many dying people are deprived of because the circumstances are not conducive to this type of death? When death becomes inevitable, is the process of dying something to experience fully? Is our fear of death a cultural distortion, an intensified fear, a false panic; do we make death worse than it really is?

Eddy told me one day that an old friend of his, who suffered from multiple handicaps and certainly did not have much time left, comforted him when she told him, "You know, Eddy, death is less frightening than you think."

Perhaps it would have been frightening if he had undergone a colostomy. Or if his family had mourned him prematurely. Or if he hadn't received sufficient pain medication.

Eddy died surrounded by an accepting, supportive family in his home and rejected the hospital environment and treatments. Eddy always claimed that his body belonged to him, and it was his privilege to do with it what he wanted.

If Eddy could have articulated what he wanted his death to teach, it would be this: Life becomes real when we approach death for the first time; otherwise life is only a dream. It was only when Eddy integrated

31

the concept of death into his life that he felt completely alive. One has not really lived until one is dying. The experience Eddy went through made him free. He was totally alive because he knew he was dying.

Given Eddy's philosophy, it would make sense to celebrate rather than mourn death. Why not sit shiva (the Jewish tradition of mourning) before rather than after someone dies? Why is the dying person alone excluded, at least in cases where he would have liked to be part of it? I do not mean that there should be joyous dancing but ceremonies with the appropriate amount of seriousness that will help the dying person feel less isolated and more alive than ever before.

As I'll discuss later in the book, Eddy's death may serve as a model for how people will die in the future.

Case 8: Robert

On a Sunday morning, my wife and I visited our friend, Robert, who was dying of generalized cancer. My wife sadly remarked that everyone is now dying of cancer, and at the end of our visit she insisted we both have a complete medical checkup. I did not find it necessary to remind her that a few months before Robert's generalized cancer had been discovered, he had had a complete checkup and was found to be in perfect health, just as our friends and relatives who died of cancer were found to be in perfect health within the year that preceded the discovery of their deadly disease.

Like many families of patients dying of cancer, Robert and his family searched for someone to blame. Typically, when I diagnose a malignancy people ask questions such as: Why didn't I recognize the malignancy in a prior checkup one year ago; or, why didn't the doctor who referred the patient to me recognize the disease in time? Like many others, it was difficult for Robert and his family to accept the inexplicable; they wanted to focus their anger on someone or some thing.

Robert underwent extensive chemotherapy during the last few months of his life, and it did not work. In fact, it made his condition worse. Robert and his family were bitter about it because the physician stopped the chemotherapy and referred him back to his family physician. Robert was still working two weeks before chemotherapy was started and four weeks after chemotherapy he was emaciated and unable to eat. He was very weak, unable to walk, barely able to speak and coughing continuously. The family believed chemotherapy was responsible for the deteriorating condition, and it's possible they were correct.

It was obvious that Robert was unhappy and even angry about the way his terminal condition had been handled by the medical profession and everyone else in general. He knew that the course of his disease was irreversible because the cancer was already widespread when it was diagnosed. He was not angry with a specific doctor or institution, but with the whole approach to a terminally ill patient. In spite of all our progress in medicine, Robert would have been better off in some isolated village without a herd of medical specialists, with just a family physician ordering the required sedation, and with his wife, children, and friends visiting from time to time.

More so than the chemotherapy, Robert's anger and frustration were making his condition worse. He hated the way he was shuttled from one specialist to another. Each one talked about a new treatment that was worse than the previous one. Each specialist sent him to another one for treatment of a specific complaint. It became a macabre and morbid merry-go-round. Finally, he looked for relief in death that would remove him from this scary and disorienting carnival ride.

What We Can Learn from Robert's Death

Death is inevitable and the ultimate goal of a full life, and no colostomy, nephrostomy, tracheotomy, or chemotherapy should interfere with it. Behind all the man-made anxieties that terminally ill patients experience, I sometimes see in their eyes a place of peace and serenity. I vaguely saw it in Robert's face. Before I saw it, I looked upon him with what could only be described as pity. But given the peace and serenity I glimpsed, maybe it was the reverse: Robert was pitying me, the one remaining. He understood, and I didn't.

I learned from Robert's case to stop lying and answer all questions honestly. I learned never to promise the patient or the family any miracle cure with chemotherapy or any other treatment and to avoid language that fostered false hope. False hope is terribly harmful because the reality of the coming death is put aside and no one is prepared for it when it must be faced. I learned to inform the family that I will answer any questions they or the patient have. Regardless of how specific and detailed the questions are, I always answer them accurately. I found that patients have a way of asking questions only if and when they can face the answer. They never ask anything they are not able to deal with, and if you do tell them something they cannot accept, they manage to block it out quickly and never ask again.

Case 9: Ms. Peters

Ms. Peters had been in charge of the Intensive Care Unit (ICU) where she had worked all her life. She was familiar with all kinds of terminal conditions such as widespread cancer, heart failure and cerebral hemorrhage. When her breast cancer was diagnosed, it had already spread to the bones and the lungs, and she had was under no illusions about the course of her disease. Since Mrs. Peters developed a bad reaction to chemotherapy and decided to discontinue it, she only required palliative treatment. She started to cough and experience difficulty in breathing. Mrs. Peters and I had managed many terminal cases and she knew my beliefs: patients should never suffer any physical pain or experience any anxiety, and they should have a good night's sleep. She knew that I favored a peaceful death over an extended one. With this in mind, she asked me to take charge of her terminal condition.

After a few days of treatment, her pain and anxiety disappeared. She started to breathe slightly better and her usual good humor returned. She even got out of bed to sit in a chair. One morning when I came to see her during my daily rounds, I noticed that something strange had happened to her. Her face wore an expression that could only be described as transcendent; her body posture was relaxed and peaceful. When she talked, I felt that this was a person who had gained some wonderful, blessed insight.

Mrs. Peters told me how she woke up in the middle of her sleep and an extraterrestrial man took her by the hand and guided her through some dark street at the end of which was a huge gate. She described the gate as the Gate of Hell of Auguste Rodin, but when it opened and she went through it, still guided by the man, she found herself in a fantastic garden which she described as the Garden of Eden. The light was magical, the music was heavenly. She met many people in this garden, some she knew as previous patients or relatives that had passed away and others she did not know. They all were in the same state of ecstasy as she, and they all welcomed her. She was completely healthy and there was no trace of cancer in her body. Without moving much, she was almost flying over the garden. Time and space were nonexistent. She finally ended up in front of another gate and was reluctant to go through it because she wanted to stay in the Garden of Eden. Her guide, always by her side, reassured her that she would eventually come back.

When she opened her eyes in the morning, she sadly found herself back in her hospital bed. She eagerly described her experience to nurses around her, but they all dismissed her story as a delirium because she kept insisting that it was real and not a dream. The resident on duty even proposed heavy sedation but she adamantly refused.

I had heard this type of dream before—a Near Death Experience (NDE). I knew that she was not delirious because in every other respect her mind was clear. I even called a psychiatrist to interview her and he declared her mind perfectly sound in every respect. I also knew that there was no drug accumulation in her body because her liver and kidneys were functioning properly and eliminating the drugs properly. Besides, the blood levels of the various drugs were within normal limits. Therefore, I did not see anything wrong with her and did not interfere with her state of euphoria. In other terminal patients who were anxious and depressed, I have tried to catalyze this euphoric state with the proper drugs. When this euphoria occurs naturally, I certainly don't interfere. NDE repeated itself for her during the following nights, although less intensely. Interestingly, her exuberance increased during the day. This situation persisted for the next five days during which she requested less and less medication; the last two days of her life she was without medication, not even for sleep. On the last day I could see that she was ready to leave this world. She died smiling, the vision of another place drawing her out of this one.

What We Can Learn from Mrs. Peters' Death

Ms. Peters was well known to many physicians who had worked with her in the ICU. Practically all of them considered her delirious due to her terminal disease. I have observed many terminal patients who were delirious, and I know that this was not the case at all. It strikes me that Mrs. Peters, like Eddy, might have possessed an understanding denied to the rest of us. As euphoric as they were, they were not out of touch with reality. Certainly the way you interpret Mrs. Peters' NDE depends on your religious convictions; some might interpret it as a glimpse of heaven.

Even if you're not religious, however, you can interpret her dream as symbolic. It represented a peaceful end to one life and the start of another journey. To her, death was a glorious moment, not a horrific one. Since no one knows what happens after we die, her dream was no more delusional than picturing a vast nothingness. Mrs. Peters chose to view the mystery one way while others choose a different vision.

Mrs. Peters' perspective strikes me as preferable, and I firmly believe that it's a perspective more of us can and should share.

Case 10: Mrs. Herman

A nurse whom I've known for more than 30 years, Mrs. Herman has always been a good-natured and dedicated professional. As the mother of three children, she's always had her hands full raising them and pursuing her career. Still, when her 61-year-old mother was diagnosed with Alzheimer's disease, she had her mom move in with her. Though at first she had tried to share the responsibility for her mother's care with her two brothers and their families, Mrs. Herman's mother preferred to be with her daughter. The demands on Mrs. Herman became so great that she had to quit her nursing job and devote herself to her mother's care full time. For six years, she shuttled her mother back-and-forth between doctor's offices, hospitals, specialty care centers and emergency rooms. The last six months of her mother's life was especially difficult, placing tremendous emotional pressure on Mrs. Herman and creating tension within her own family. When her mother died, she left her modest estate to her daughter, but the will was contested by her brothers, creating a rift that has never healed.

Then Mrs. Herman's mother-in-law had a cerebral hemorrhage and was partially paralyzed and in need of care. Mr. Herman felt that they should give his mother the same care as his wife's mother received, so his mother moved into their home. For the next eight years, it was a repeat of the nightmare with Mrs. Herman's mother. By the time she died of a heart attack, the demands of her care and the associated emotional issues had taken their toll. Mrs. Herman's children found the environment especially excruciating.

The two oldest children left home, then the youngest daughter moved out when she turned 18. Mrs. Herman and her husband divorced two years later.

Today, Mrs. Herman has returned to her nursing career but she still bears the scars of her experiences. She talks obsessively about old people who live too long and is bitter about having sacrificed so much of her life to take care of her mother who lived for years as a prisoner of her own deteriorated mind; she also complained about her mother-in-law who kept telling everyone who would listen, I want to die and I don't want anyone to take care of me. Mrs. Herman was especially angry at the medical establishment for extending lives that no one wants extended.

What We Can Learn From Mrs. Herman's Experiences:

Taking care of a disabled and dying loved one is a job that no one is really prepared for. It's easy to underestimate the toll it takes both in terms of time commitment and emotional upheaval. Certainly Mrs. Herman's case is extreme, in that she had to endure the same horrific situation twice and that it went on for a combined total of 14 years. Still, it points up how many adult children feel when they try and care for a dying parent. There's tremendous anger not only at healthcare professionals who are extending life past all reasonable limits but at dying parents for demanding so much of their children.

The lesson here is that we need to listen to the request for death of Mrs. Herman's mother-in-law rather than extending life in defiance of that request. We should also learn that bringing a dying loved one home can be an emotional time bomb in a family; that family members need to deal with their own feelings about death before embarking on this journey.

A COMMON THEME

In the ten stories I've related here, fear is a word that frequently emerges in the narrative. It's not only the dying patient who is afraid, but the family, friends and medical staff. It's not enough to admit that everyone is afraid of death and that it's an inevitable part of the process. Too often, the fear is blinding. It prevents us from seeing that our last months and moments on earth can be fulfilling rather than frightening; it causes us to treat dying people as some odd and alien species.

We need to address the issue of our fear of death: what causes it, why it's so overpowering, how we might lessen it and turn it into something else. The next chapter will explore this issue in detail.

Chapter 3

FEAR OF DEATH

We did not come here to stay. Everything in life reminds us about death. ... Eulogy

We have it within our power to make death a much better experience than it currently is. Better is a relative term. It can mean less painful. It can also translate as more fulfilling, a fitting conclusion to a well-lived life. A better death might also be interpreted as everything from faster to more dignified.

Unfortunately, a number of obstacles stand in the way of this better death. Legal, social and medical issues all have set up barriers, and we'll discuss them in ensuing chapters. But there's another, less tangible barrier that we've erected, and it comes from our ignorance. We do not understand death very well. Certainly we have a grasp of what the process entails—most of us have experienced the death of a loved one or a good friend—but we don't view it holistically.

What we need to do is see it within a different and much broader context. Until we do, we'll harbor misconceptions and be vulnerable to myths. The goal of this chapter is to provide a context, starting with the contrast between human and animal death.

What is a Natural Death?

When animals die in the wild, they die differently than humans in hospitals, hospices or homes. The three differentiating characteristics are:

· **Death occurs at or near full maturity (rather than in old age)**
Animals usually die near or at the peak of their physical strength. All it takes is a slight defect—a thorn stuck deep in a paw, an abscessed tooth—and they starve to death or become easy prey. An antelope that loses speed, a bird that cannot fly and a fish that can't swim fast enough

are condemned.

· **It is rapid (the pre-death period is not artificially extended)**
Typically, a rapid animal death involves violence. They may suffer intensely—picture a wildebeest being ravaged by a pack of dogs—but the suffering is brief. Even animals that are starving tend not to die of starvation per se but at the hands of predators who observe the weakened condition of their victims.

· **There's no consciousness of dying (they do not feel, meditate on or agonize about the event)**
Animals have no consciousness whatsoever. While this is an arguable point, most would agree that if consciousness exists, it's quite primitive. Unlike the human brain, the animal brain has no independence; it cannot think, reflect, ponder or grasp the concepts of life and death. Animals experience pain and thus they scream when they are torn apart by a predator's jaws. But when animals are killed by barbiturate injection, they react calmly (as do other animals witnessing this event). They lack the consciousness necessary to react the way a human would.

Once upon a time—perhaps two or three million years ago—these animal death traits were shared by humans. Though human evolution has changed the way we experience death, we retain traces of these animal characteristics. Sometimes, there are more than traces. Regressive behaviors can lead to regressive deaths. The phrase, He died like a dog , can be taken both literally and figuratively.

Still, human death is, in a way, opposite animal death. There are differences—the flip sides of the three animal death traits:

· **Our extended lifespan.** Dying of old age is a new evolutionary wrinkle.

· **The slowness of the process.** We die day by day, week by week, year by year from diseases and general debilitation. The pain and suffering may be less intense, but it's dragged out far longer.

· **Our intense awareness of death.** This is what makes us so afraid of dying.

Given these traits, what is a natural death? Is it death in full maturity or in old age? Is it more natural to die quickly and violently in the jaws of a predator, or connected to machines for months in a hospital? Is our consciousness of dying natural, or is it more natural to exist in the anxiety-free state of an animal? These are issues we'll discuss in detail in later chapters. For now, however, it's important to start thinking about them. We need to set the stage for a discussion of what's a natural death versus what's a preferable death.

WHY THE LAWS OF NATURE ARE NOT THE LAWS OF MAN

From an evolutionary perspective, natural selection looks perfect. According to Charles Darwin, survival of the fittest is the process by which those with superior qualities are chosen to survive and reproduce while those who are less fit are rejected.

While the process is perfect from a pragmatic standpoint, it is also clumsy, wasteful, blundering, low and horribly cruel... Or so said Charles Darwin. Perhaps he was aghast that between 90 and 99.9 percent of a given species must perish before they reach maturity and the ability to reproduce. Or it might be that he found it cruel that many who were selected by nature to reproduce die as soon as they can no longer reproduce.

Of course, the natural death of those who cease to reproduce is cruel only by human standards. Nature has no use for old age. It has no time, space or resources to spare. It wants to clear out the old and make room for the new. This is the type of death that we inherited from our animal ancestry.

As human beings, our impulse is to take nature to task. Over billions of years, nature has improved and perfected almost every human organ and function. From our care of progeny to our cardiac pulmonary vascular systems to our mode of locomotion, we've evolved splendidly.

41

It is therefore appalling that nature has not perfected a mode of dying for humans; that it has, in fact, made dying far worse for humans than animals. As an obstetrician, I can appreciate the brilliant job nature has done with our reproduction system. But as a physician who has cradled many dying patients in his arms, I am outraged by the shoddy work done on the human dying process. It is as if nature put all its effort in perfecting our entry into the world and, exhausted from such a mammoth task, did a quick and sloppy job in planning our exit.

If one is religious, one can blame God for this oversight, I suppose. I prefer to blame nature. I cannot believe that God, in His infinite wisdom and love for mankind, could have chosen that we die in the way we do. In either case, the conclusion is obvious: Our deaths are not natural or, at least, not perfect.

That's not to say that death itself is not natural and necessary. Without it, we would have a nightmarishly overpopulated and truly barbaric world. But we are usually denied a happy death, one in which we go to sleep peacefully and don't wake up. This type of happy death is rare because, from a medical standpoint, we automatically wake up when a life threatening condition occurs during sleep. It's a terrible thing to write, but if we could foresee the agony of our deaths, some of us might wish we were never born. If we could see into our futures, we might witness ourselves, our families, our doctors and our lawyers mismanaging our dying. Given this vision, we certainly would end our lives just before this terrible process commenced.

Consider a disturbing definition of death: a hybrid of animal death and human interference.

The Evolution of Death

Many of us think about death inflexibly. Certain habits, rituals and attitudes have become ingrained, and we resist new perspectives. Part of the problem is that we can't see far enough back into the past to realize that our approach to death is relatively new; that in pre-history there were other ways of looking at the process. Based on my studies, I've determined that death evolved in five stages:

Stage 1: From the beginning of life on earth about a half billion years ago to the appearance of the first pre-humans (Homo Erectus) about 1.2 millions years ago, death was animal-like.

Stage 2: From 1.2 million years ago to about 50,000 years ago when Neanderthals disappeared and archaic Homo Sapiens appeared, there was an increased awareness of death and concern about an afterlife. Old age, though probably uncommon, must have been met with hostility, and disposal of the old and the sick must have been dreaded. This dread can be glimpsed in the practices of earlier generations of Eskimos and Pacific Islanders.

Stage 3: As Homo Sapiens flourished, old age became more common but was still considered a terrible thing. Unless old people were good storytellers or possessed some skill, they were viewed with hostility; old people were unproductive and therefore a burden. It is likely that elderly people suffered greatly.

Stage 4: During the modern era, elderly people (or senior citizens, a label that clearly distinguishes them from others) exist as a group apart; they have their own rights and depend less on others. Old people spend much of their time fearfully, desperately and often unsuccessfully searching for an extended life and a satisfactory death.

Stage 5: This stage of a better death is yet to come, hopefully.

Most of us cannot see beyond or behind Stage 4. Attitudes have hardened, and all of us resist any change in the way we view old age and death. Doctors often become hostile when it's suggested that they should not employ extraordinary means to keep someone alive; patients leave orders and families insist that the plug not be pulled even if there isn't a chance that patients can be revived.

Though these narrow attitudes stem in part from our being unable to view death from an evolutionary perspective, they also arise from our unwillingness to face our fear of death.

FACING THE FEAR OF DEATH

Our fear of death is the price we humans pay for our awareness of being alive. People who are truly unafraid of dying are psychologically sick; they will probably end up dying in a stupid and meaningless way. The delusion that there is nothing to fear will send them jumping off bridges or trying some death-defying stunt. Like someone who can feel no pain, they receive no warning signals that might prevent them from risking and losing their lives.

Fear of death is inevitable and omnipresent. Even if we're in perfect health, we worry about it. Even when we sleep, we dream about it. Some of us are so afraid of the concept that we can't bear to talk about death. Even though we reject the notion or try and block our thoughts about dying, they invariably creep into our consciousness.

On a first approach, there is nothing neurotic or abnormal in our fear of death. People are naturally terrified of the unknown, of what happens to them after they die. The experiences of being in contact with terminal patients bring this fear into sharp relief. Common fears and tortured paradoxes expressed by people who are dying include:

Falling asleep terrified they won't wake up, and if they do wake up worrying that this the last time they will wake up.

Being able to perceive the world yet panic-stricken at the thought that soon their perceptions will end.

Desperately wanting to relate to other people but no longer wishing to relate to anyone.

Feeling one's lungs breathing and heart beating but knowing that these organs will soon cease to function.

The intense anxiety these thoughts and feelings generate may have as much to do with a patient's death as the disease itself. As we'll discuss later on, anxiety-relieving drugs might help these patients a great deal, but they're usually not used to the extent that they should be. As a result, the dying and even the elderly are living their own deaths. Ironically, it is the intensity of life—of being conscious, emotional and human—that makes death so terrifying.

Despite all this, many people don't acknowledge their fear is constant and real. Instead, they ignore, rationalize and deny it. Or they trust in God and the promise of an afterlife to alleviate their fears. Others face death with great courage, repressing their fears in the name of a higher cause—they become heroes of one sort or another. Yet even for those who bury their fear of death to the depth of the unconscious mind, the reality is that they are as frightened as anyone.

The fear of death is not necessarily harmful and sometimes serves a purpose. Life can become overwhelming, and most people at one point or another have difficulty coping with the stress. If it were not for the fear, suicide would be much more tempting and commonplace than it is.

We aren't born with this fear; it develops along with our consciousness. Infants and small children don't fear death; they may react to and fear pain, but that isn't the same thing. They don't care about dying because they don't grasp the concept of life. It's only when we realize what it is to be alive that we start being afraid of dying.

Rationally, we know that we have to die eventually; that the world would become uninhabitable without death; that death is a natural process far preferable to being a vegetable. But, the fear of death is irrational, which is why it's a mistake to try and reason a person out of his fear of death. Still, there are therapeutic and even religious approaches that view fear of death as abnormal and attempt to relieve that fear through logical argument.

We can trace this fear back to the rise of consciousness thousands of years ago. When we started to become thinking, feeling beings, we began to seek rational explanations for every significant event that touched our lives:

Will the sun rise tomorrow like it did today?
Will winter end?

Will people wake up after they go to sleep?
What happens after you die?

Unfortunately, there is no rational answer to the last question. If death could be explained logically, we could alleviate our fears.

THE MANY FACES OF FEAR:

Let's get to the heart of our fear of death. I've had many patients talk about the desirability of a quick and painless death. They don't seem to have much fear of dying from a heart attack in their sleep; they also endorse euthanasia as a preferable alternative. What really chills their blood, however, is the passage from life to death. Contemplating that passage is terrifying; contemplating a quick and painless exit is not as terrifying.

Many people's fear takes on an obsessive tone as they continuously ask questions such as:

When am I going to die?
How will I die?
Will I be incapacitated?
Will I suffer?
Who will take care of me when I'm sick and dying?
Will I still be able to take care of myself?

This anxious questioning of impending death becomes agonizing. It's not worry about the physical pain associated with the passage as much as the emotional and mental suffering that arises because death is inevitable and there is nothing one can do to prevent it.

Two other realities contribute to our fear of death and uniquely human responses to it:

· People die in relative isolation.

· Humans surrounding a dying person interfere with the process of death.

As we'll see, we can control many of these factors in ways that lessen people's fears but we frequently fail to do so.

What will be continuously stressed in this manuscript is the distinction between: 1) the eventuality of death, which is more or less accepted by everyone; 2) the process of dying, which is tremendously feared in view of the pain and anxiety associated with it. The first one is natural death and nothing can be done about it. The second, however, is the result of our evolutionary and cultural process and is man-made. This book is about what we can do regarding the latter and how we can re-create the process in a more modern, humane manner.

Chapter 4

THE SUCCESSIVE STAGES OF THE DYING PROCESS

"The load was getting heavy and God closed his weary eyes."
–Old Negro Spiritual

After closely following the deaths of more than one hundred patients, I classified their deaths into different stages. To a certain extent, this classification is presumptuous; each death is personal and unique. Still, we can distinguish certain feelings and behaviors that are common to many deaths, and they form an evolutionary pattern that is unmistakable. Some of these stages may overlap; their order may change; one or more stages may be skipped; and some dying patients may become stuck in any of these stages.

Patients who are dying fall into two categories: those who know they are dying and those who do not. This is not a clean distinction. At some level of his conscious or unconscious mind, almost every dying patient registers the fact that the end is near. Over the weeks or even months that precede death, most people become familiar with the fact that death is irreversible. They usually go through the following successive stages:

First Stage: Complete Denial.
Death is completely rejected and hidden in the unconscious mind. Dying patients go on with life as usual and may stay at this stage until the end. They have no conscious knowledge of their coming death, although in their dreams or in some deep level of their unconscious mind they sense it. They know they are sick, even seriously sick, but they are confident that they are just going through a difficult time and will eventually recover. They may die suddenly or sink into a coma.

Denial is common in relatively young people, but it can be encountered at any age. These individuals can be of any social or educational level and approximately ten percent of dying patients become stuck in this stage. Most block everything from their minds during the time preceding death. The surrounding people are left with the impression that the patient died not knowing he was dying. Friends and family usually consider this the happiest way to die and do anything they can to make sure the dying patient is unaware of the coming death. I've seen patients die very slowly yet never give any indication that they understand they're dying. Sometimes the patients are attempting to reassure the living, pretending to be doing fine so they don't have to deal with other people's grief. They may even turn the tables and request reassurance from family and friends that I'm doing better. They talk about their future lives as if death were not a foregone conclusion. They learn the questions not to ask and who not to ask them of, tiptoeing around the reality of death.

It is unbelievable how far this denial can go. I knew patients who were told that their cancer had spread to the liver and to the lungs; others were told that their widespread cancer had not responded to any treatment. Yet some of these patients talked about and made plans for the future as if they were going to have a long life ahead of them. I am of the opinion that the denial patient hears only what he wants and completely blocks out the rest. Patients are receptive only to what they are capable of receiving. No matter what a doctor tells them about their condition, they filter out the news they cannot tolerate.

Patients in denial sometimes share certain traits. They have lived a life without excitement or any highly emotional event. War veterans or Holocaust survivors, for instance, would never deny a coming death. People in denial also rarely talk about death; they do not visit or comment on a dying patient. Their lives have been unadventurous in many respects. The process of dying is just too much for them to deal with and they mobilize all their energy to ignore it.

Second Stage: Fighting Death.

The patient realizes that he may die and courageously fights the disease. He accepts and willingly cooperates with any and all treatments regardless of how complicated, painful, useless, or even harmful they might be. Hope keeps people fighting. When they finally die, they are praised for their courage and determination to battle the disease to the bitter end and for never giving up hope. As perplexing as this fighting attitude is, it means that people fail to accept death. About 10 to 15 percent of patients freeze at this level and fight to the end.

This stage is actually more prevalent among the people surrounding the dying patient than the actual patient. When a well-known person is dying of cancer, the news media covers it extensively. Family members and even doctors comment on the determination and courage of the sick patient. But during my entire career of dealing with terminal patients, I never heard of or saw a patient fighting the disease to the bitter end. When I used to question this fight, friends and relatives of the dying patient would become angry with me. If I were to suggest that a treatment was futile, I was looked upon as an heretic. The people surrounding the patient acted as if the fight was a holy war, a crusade against threatening death, and that I was some kind of traitor because I refused to endorse it. I've learned not to question the value of fighting death or to mention that the private interests of a whole industry depends on fighting death to the bitter end.

Third Stage: Fear.

Panic is an early and visible symptom of this fear. The surrounding circle of family, friends, acquaintances, nurses, and doctors dread this stage; they are as afraid as the patient. As a result, they transfer their own fear to the patient, often making him more afraid than he would ordinarily be. Though the patient rarely becomes stuck at this stage, the surrounding people often do. As the dying person moves on to the next stage, he may leave family and even medical personnel behind as he evolves toward death.

This third group, almost half of all dying patients, is definitely the largest. The patient knows he is dying, and all the family and friends know it, too.

Some patients who know they are dying manipulate the surrounding family by screaming, "Don't you know I am dying!" and the family, frightened by the idea that the patient is going to break the taboo, immediately complies with whatever request the patient makes. Some dying patients are adroit at using their deaths as a threat. Unless family or medical staff meet their requests, they will verbalize the fact of their dying. This can be intimidating and result in people doing all sorts of inappropriate and even bizarre things for people who are dying.

Some people in this third group know that a member (or members) of the surrounding family cannot cope with the idea of seeing them dying. Although a patient would be relieved if they discussed his coming death, they refrain from doing so thinking they'll spare him that pain. Patients also submit to all kinds of useless treatments to satisfy the family's wishes and allow them to believe they are doing everything possible.

I cannot stress enough that what makes this stage the most prevalent and most difficult is the behavior of the surrounding people. No longer able to deny that death is coming, they wildly vent their panic. They don't realize that it is their own panic, falsely assuming that the terminal patient is the one in a state of panic. The dying person, sensing panic around him, panics too. When death finally comes, everyone realizes how artificial the panic was and returns to their normal state of mind.

The dying patient rarely freezes at this stage; he quickly moves to the next one. The apprehension expressed by dying patients is due in part to the apprehension of family and friends who often hold the dying person at this stage.

To avoid the fear and anxiety associated with this stage, families resort to useless, expensive, and prolonged hospitalization; they call specialists and super-specialists to deal with various complaints; they bitterly criticize doctors and hospital personnel for their callousness; they involve anyone who offers a suggestion in the patient's management. Rather than dealing with this fear, families find all sorts of unproductive ways to distract themselves from it.

Fourth Stage: Limited and Shared Knowledge.

In this stage, death's approach is acknowledged and accepted by everyone, the dying person as well as the surrounding family. But not all the family members accept it readily and or not all are strong enough to discuss it openly with the dying patient. This is just as well because emotions are tense and people can take only so much. As a result, different types of communications are established between the dying person on one side and various family members on the other.

The split-knowledge patient shares information about his dying selectively. He may confide only in one person, leaving others in the dark. These private conversations usually are held with a religious minister, sometimes with the spouse and rarely with a grown son or daughter who will become responsible for the family. In a few instances, I have found myself carrying on different conversations with the dying patient and a spouse (or other family member) because the latter had been kept in the dark. In one instance, I was a messenger between a dying husband and his wife since they could not discuss the subject of wills.

Forbidden knowledge patients, on the other hand, want to discuss their death and dying openly with family members; they are eager to help the family be less panic-stricken and more accepting of death. This discussion, however, is forbidden by a family member—usually the spouse. As a result, the patient dies in isolation, having been deprived of sharing these final thoughts and feelings. This occurs frequently, and I know of many cases in which the dying person would have been relieved had free communication been established.

Open discussion about death is becoming more common, but many people shy away from it because they believe it's too cruel to the dying patient. In reality, it's compassionate rather than cruel, and the anxiety produced by open discussion is often in family members. A dying patient's anxiety is often relieved by such discussion. Hopefully, with more education, the circle of these discussions will widen.

Fifth Stage: Peaceful Acceptance.

This is the stage where the knowledge that death is soon to come is freely communicated between the terminal patient and the surrounding people—family, friends, religious ministers, treating personnel. Death is now accepted, and it is often accepted calmly. Not that there is always free and open discussion, but the fact of the coming death is well understood and accepted. The role of the medical profession and other healthcare personnel is diminished. Any proposed treatment is fully discussed in terms of advantages and disadvantages and more often than not it is turned down. What is now important for the physician is to relieve physical pain and prescribe medication for a good night's sleep; no more heroic measures for a fight to the bitter end. The family and dying individual are able to discuss disposal of assets, making a will, a living will, plans for the future of the family to be left behind, and even funeral ceremony and burial.

More dying patients reach this stage than you might think, and many more could reach it if the circumstances were right. Unfortunately, the medical profession does not help patients reach this stage despite the fact that people increasingly recognize the importance of acceptance and demand doctors help them achieve it.

Sometimes patients accept death alone, while the surrounding people are usually stuck in any of the first four stages. It's difficult to identify one explanation for why people accept death. Some see no purpose in fighting death to the bitter end. Others are just tired of the increasingly difficult struggle to stay alive. I've had patients who feel they are useless, a burden and even an imposition on their families. There are also some people who feel that death is a natural and inevitable process one has to go through.

As unusual as it might seem, some patients resist the idea of reversing the death process. They don't want to stay alive for an additional few months or even be cured by a new treatment. They hate the notion of having to start the process of dying all over again at some point in the near future. Almost uniformly, patients explain why they turn down these death-reversing treatments with the following reasoning:

The process of dying is a long journey that is difficult to start, and they may as well finish it. One is going to die anyway, so why not now?

Sixth Stage: The Cosmic Death.

Evolving to this stage is rare. It's a stage in which the dying process is ecstatic, positive and illuminating. Although this joyous death is unusual, it is present to some degree in many dying patients. It would become more obvious and occur more frequently if people were allowed to express it and if pain were completely relieved. This ecstatic death is euphoric, reflecting the Cabalist prayer for the dead: "Come death, oh beautiful bride!" In the rare situations where patients have reached this stage, friends, family and even doctors are frightened. They don't understand the patient's ecstatic calm.

In an ecstatic death, the dying patient is intensely *living* the dying process. Paradoxically, the patient's feelings are often hidden because he withdraws from and barely communicates with surrounding people to avoid frightening them. The patient simply belongs to another world and considers himself already dead. As you can imagine, it is very difficult for the dying patient to describe this feeling. We lack a language or other mode of communication between the living and the near dead at this stage.

While it's rare for patients to die in this stage, it's not at all unusual for them to experience some aspect of it. We routinely see dying people who experience moments of great joy and contentment. These moments, however, are fleeting. The surrounding family is so terrified by this incomprehensible (to them) reaction that they become visibly upset or confused, and this causes the patient to retreat to an earlier, more acceptable stage of dying.

This ecstatic mode of death has been extensively described by people who thought they had died of a serious disease or injury, but were revived either temporarily or permanently. This Near Death Experience (NDE) is extensively described in modern literature (*The Light Beyond*, R.A. Moody, Jr., M.D.; *Saved by the Light*, D. Brinkley; *Heading Toward*

Omega, K. Ring, among many others). NDE is a kind of glimpse of Heaven, that has been described by people who thought they were dying and for all practical purposes, died. This is a very common experience, especially today when many patients go through major surgery or recover from a severe heart attack. I have observed this experience many times. I have also observed it in terminal patients, as reported in a previous chapter (Eddy, Case #7 and Mrs. Peters, Case #9). It is quite possible that people who die experience the same euphoric feelings. I will report later on how it can be induced in terminal patients through the use of specific drugs.

The last two stages, peaceful acceptance and cosmic death, are unique and specific to the dying patient and are rarely experienced by the people surrounding the dying patient. Feeling pity, compassion or even sorrow for those who are dying seems absurd, given that they are in blissful states. *Ars moriendi*, the art of dying, is something all of us need to understand and learn so that we don't react to or manage a person's death in inappropriate and harmful ways.

SUBJECTIVE AND OBJECTIVE DEATH

"To be or not to be, that is the question."

Within these six stages, there are some common attitudes and perceptions that we should now examine.

Solipsism is the notion that nothing exists outside of the self. In other words, an individual believes that if he dies, the universe dies with him. In a sense, this is the ultimate ego trip; we are the center of the universe and it has been created only for us. This is an attribute of consciousness and it can be a powerful driving force when we are alive and active. Death is dreaded, however, when, during the process of dying we realize we are not the center of the universe and that the universe will continue without us. Even worse, after the universe has incorporated the fruits of our labor, it can do just fine without us.

I refer to this mindset as subjective because it's highly personal and self-centered. People feel what matters is that they are dying and will no longer perceive the world, and they have very little interest in how the universe will continue after they're gone. I have seen cases where a dying person who had been socially responsible and a loving, caring family member suddenly had no concern whatsoever about what would happen to friends and family after his death; apres moi, le deluge (after me, the flood).

The opposite approach to death is more objective and realistic. In these cases, dying people understand that they will no longer perceive the universe subjectively but that it will continue existing and be perceived by others. Their feelings for and thoughts about their world will be gone, but feelings and thoughts will still be experienced by others in that world. They recognize that everything will stay the same after their death, and they are only one tiny event of the universe. This emotional and intellectual release of the universe is crucial for accepting this objective concept of death. A friend of mine, whom I once consulted about writing a will to take care of my family after my death, told me, "After you are dead, the world will look different." Once we release the world to its objective existence and stop perceiving it subjectively, it is indeed very much different.

UNCONSCIOUS RECEPTIVITY TO DEATH

There is something within us ready to accept death, something that *only* people in the process of dying become aware of.

The unconscious mind may be aware of and receptive to death as it approaches long before the conscious mind registers it. It's a misconception that our unconscious mind produces terrifying nightmares when death is near. Dying patients usually sleep quietly and peacefully. It is the conscious mind that often is terrified of death. The unconscious mind often embraces death, accepting the end peacefully. Deep within us, we naturally move toward death as a way out, as a natural and normal ending of life and as a part of life. The unconscious mind is not bound by any of our social or cultural norms, something that people in good health have difficulty comprehending.

The unconscious mind may register awareness of coming death while the conscious mind does not. The conscious mind, unreceptive to the idea of death, may block it. For some people, this can be beneficial if they're not ready to face death. When patients are not ready, they rationalize themselves out of it, block it and forget it, no matter how clearly the facts of their medical condition are communicated. The Ego and Mechanism of Defense (Freud S, 1967) and The Ego and Mechanism Adaptation (Freud A, 1972) are informative about how the conscious ego represses the idea of death.

Not to be aware of coming death, however, is only skin deep. This subconscious or unconscious awareness manifests itself in all kinds of ways. Like Eddy (Case #7) in our case history chapter, one can say that we are born with the seed of death or death instinct.

STANDING IN THE WAY OF DEATH

A living creature is a mixture of living and dying processes. When we are vibrant with life, the living process is dominant, but, when we are aging or dying, the process of death takes over. We naturally transition to the death process; difficult life conditions or a severe disease that lasts too long are all it takes to spawn a death wish. If it were not for the fear of suffering, the interference of the surrounding people and the exquisite terror of not knowing what happens to the soul after death, the wish to die would be more frequently expressed.

During a recent hospital Mortality Review Committee session, a young attending physician from the Department of Medicine expressed his dismay about the DNR (do not resuscitate) orders signed by an increasing number of patients—more than half the patients today sign such a request. This young physician had been trained to use any and all lifesaving procedures regardless of the advanced age of the patient and the advanced status of a terminal disease. I knew that this doctor saw himself as a God-like figure, employing heroic measures to keep patients alive for a few additional hours or days. When he employed these measures, he refrained from mentioning to the usually distraught family the tremendous pain that was the tradeoff for a few hours or days of additional life.

Like many younger doctors, this one was upset about the rise in

DNR orders because he had little understanding of death and dying. He is probably also perturbed that a growing number of dying patients and their families are rejecting interventional procedures that do more harm than good. This young doctor can deal only with the reality of life because he was never trained in the reality of death. He is not aware of it, does not know how to treat it, he denies it and ultimately harms his patients. As we'll see it in the next chapter, the entire healthcare community needs to learn a better, more humane way to manage the process of dying.

Chapter 5

MISMANAGEMENT OF DYING PATIENTS

Who is in charge of a dying patient?

The management of terminally ill patients has always been approached negatively in Western society, but we seem to be moving from negativity to insanity. It is not an exaggeration to write that almost every dying patient who reaches the emergency room of any hospital is automatically subjected to unbelievable tortures. Little if any explanation is given to the patient regarding the nature of the condition or the futility of the torturous interventional procedures.

Certainly every once in a great while these procedures result in a miraculous recovery or add quality months or years to someone's life. On the rare occasions when these miracles happen, there's a great deal of positive publicity about what was done, making it seem like these miracles happen every day. What isn't publicized is the frequent failure of these procedures and the additional suffering imposed on many patients.

No One is in Charge

Everyone has a say in how terminally ill patients should be treated but no one has the final say. In other words, it's a participatory process where everyone involved is under the illusion that another participant is in charge. In reality, patients, family, friends, healthcare professionals, hospital administrators and religious figures all assume that someone else is responsible for making key decisions. Let's look at the mindset of each of these groups and how they fail to take responsibility or are prevented from doing so.

As unbelievable as it seems, the dying patient has practically no say in the way he should be treated. Besides, the patient's ability to take charge is limited by his fears and personal problems as well as his lack of knowledge about what's happening to him. Most patients possess only a vague idea of the prognosis, and everyone is afraid to discuss the coming death with these patients. As a result, dying people have little ability to evaluate the proposed procedure. I have no quarrel with those who refuse to tell patients the truth. When dealing with terminally ill patients during my career, I was brutally honest only with the consent of the family and when I thought patients could handle it. When I did tell patients the truth, however, they never reacted hysterically or committed suicide. Interestingly, the truth produced hysteria only in people surrounding the dying patient. The truth, when requested by dying patients, often helped them achieve a sense of peace.

The family is not in charge because they are acting on irrational (though heartfelt) impulses. Because they will soon lose a loved one, they communicate their despair in the dying patient's presence, making him feel guilty for dying and causing them so much pain. Consequently, he goes along with the family members' wishes to prolong the patient's life, even if all it does is buy that patient a few additional days or weeks of agony. Though the family could manage and relieve this agony, they don't; they're irrationally focused on the quantity rather than the quality of the time remaining for the patient. What families often fail to realize is that their emotions are reflected in the dying patient. "The Death Chamber," by Edvard Munch eloquently expresses this truth. In the painting, one cannot detect any difference in the facial expression of the dying patient and the family members. If family members would come to terms with their loved one's dying, they would not cause their loved ones such distress and they would be able to make more rational, humane decisions.

I have observed friends of people who are dying, and they tend to add confusion rather than wisdom to the management process. While they are in a better position than family to be rational and they certainly care about their dying friends, they often get caught up in anger—they make negative comments about the hospital staff or the way family members are treating the dying person. Rather than doing everything possible to make the dying person comfortable and content as he is dying, they get sidetracked on issues such as calling in another specialist (as if there were some magical specialist who could rescind the death sentence).

Perhaps the most common assumption is that healthcare professionals are in charge of the dying process. While they conceivably know more about the technical aspects of the process than others, their knowledge is often limited. Even worse, their authority is limited and their judgment is colored by the demands placed on them by family members. Do something! the family screams or begs, and many times doctors bow to this pressure, knowing that what they'll do won't help the patient get better and might make him feel worse. It's important to point out that just because someone is a physician, he may not be mature enough to deal with a dying patient, especially if he is in a sort of figurative denial about a patient's impending death. The role of the medical profession in managing the care of dying patients is a complex issue that I'll discuss in more detail later in the chapter.

Death is not a selling point for hospitals, and they often try and distance themselves from dying patients in a variety of ways. Administrators don't want the negative statistics that come with too many people dying under their watch. Though hospitals certainly have the human and technical resources to set up programs that manage the dying process in a humanistic manner, they rarely do so. I've seen hospitals shy away from admitting terminally ill patients; some institutions even initiate covert policies to divert terminal patients to other facilities.

Religious figures may have participated in the management of death in the past, but today the clergy has practically stopped dealing with dying patients. They rarely visit a dying patient and most of the time, the minister shows up after the patient is dead. Time after time, people delay calling in the clergy because to do so means that one accepts that the patient is about to die and for doctors and family members, this is heresy. At best, what occurs among Catholics is a private confession between priest and patient, although both parties pretend that the visit is little more than a routine social call. Too often, the role of clergy is limited to comforting the family after the death and praising the virtues of the departed at the funeral service.

The result of all this is tragic miscommunication as a patient's life is ending. The doctor falsely assumes that he is receiving directions from the patient (and the family) to keep the patient alive at all costs. The family and the patient assume that the doctor is an expert in the art and science of death and dare not interfere for fear they'll harm the patient or cause a premature death. Everyone assumes the patient is unable to make any decisions because death has somehow unhinged his mind. The hospital assumes that they are vulnerable to accusations of mismanagement and even lawsuits if they interfere in the process. Because of these false assumptions, everyone is confused and aggravated as death approaches.

These false assumptions have their root in our culture's denial of death's existence. We forget that death is inevitable. We do not consider ourselves mortal but immortal. It is ironic that death certificates in the USA (only in the USA, as far as I know) do not include natural causes as a cause of death. A few days ago, I heard the following report on the radio: Dr. Benjamin Spock, well-known pediatrician, has died at the age of 94. The cause of death has not yet been determined. That a patient could die of a naturally progressive and irreversible disease or of old age is not part of the American psyche. We firmly believe that one dies of something; that every death could have been prevented if only the right thing were done.

In this state of denial, inappropriate people and professions step in and indirectly take change of how we die. More often than not, the groups who have the greatest influence on the process of dying are the media, lawyers and extremists.

How Others Impose Their Viewpoints and Interests

Health, dying, and death are emotionally charged issues, and it's inevitable that the media will cover these issues extensively and even sensationally. Many times, this coverage has resulted in healthcare improvements; stories have pointed out deficiencies in care and treatment and have produced positive changes, including changes in the management of dying patients. At the same time, however, the media has also raised expectations of dying patient care and treatment to absurd levels. The implication of many stories is that someone is always to blame when a patient dies; it suggests that death is always unnatural. Rather than correcting the growing belief that all of us should be healthy all of the time, they reinforce it.

There is nothing healthcare professionals can do to meet the expectations raised by the media. What tends to happen, however, is that hospitals and doctors react defensively to all the horror stories and media accusations, especially when it comes to managing the care of dying patients. Consequently, they continue the tradition of unnecessary procedures and patient suffering. No one wants to take the chance and ease a patient's pain, fearing accusations of overmedicating. No one wants to contribute to a quick, peaceful death for fear of being called another Kevorkian.

The legal system contributes to this problem in similar ways. Again, lawyers have filed worthwhile medical malpractice suits that have catalyzed policies and procedures of benefit to patients. The other side of the coin, however, is that the health of patients can be compromised because their standard of care is dictated by the legal profession. In certain instances, dying patients are treated out of fear of legal consequence as well as for their condition and comfort. Every imaginable procedure that a doctor or hospital could be accused of not performing is automatically imposed on the patient, even if it creates great suffering, prolongs an agonized life or involves great expense. Without any standards for treating dying patients, fear of malpractice lawsuits can influence care.

I know a radiologist whose fear of missing any diagnosis when reading x-ray films is so great that he always lists in his reports all pathological conditions even remotely associated with what he sees or thinks he sees on the x-ray films. The treating physician, on receiving these reports, feels legally obligated to order extensive testing with numerous procedures to rule out each and every possibility. Most of these procedures are unnecessary and could be ruled out by simple clinical judgment.

Extremists also play a role in how we manage the dying process. On the one hand, there are people who are virulently anti-death. They are often the family and friends of dying patients who will fight to prolong life past any rational or logical limit. I know of parents who sold their homes or made extensive loans to take their dying child to a foreign country to visit a so-called miracle worker. I have seen a sizable inheritance depleted for the useless treatment of an older parent with widespread cancer. These people will cajole, threaten and connive in order to get medical personnel to do their bidding. No logical argument or medical facts will stop them; they're fanatical about trying to wrest every additional ounce of life from a patient, no matter what the human cost might be. The do-battle-with-death impulse might be noble in theory, but in practice it frequently results in excessive pain and suffering.

On the other end of the spectrum, there are those who consider it a sacrilege to interfere with any natural process, including death. These extremists include Jehovah's Witnesses who refuse blood transfusions, parents who do not allow their children to be vaccinated, or a woman in obstructed labor who would rather die than have a cesarean section that will save her life as well as the child's life. They are so doctrinaire in their thinking that they refuse to adapt their views to fit reality.

The problem with extremists is that they are so vociferous and uncompromising in their beliefs. They are often loud, aggressive, and will go to any length to impose their views, even if not shared by the majority. Some of these people are well-organized and part of groups that make their presence felt. It doesn't take much in our politically correct society to influence a decision in a touchy area. I've seen hospitals and doctors bow to the wishes of extremists just because of what they feared these extremists might do (rather than what they actually did). Just the thought of a public confrontation, an angry phone call to the head of the hospital or the combined might of extremists, lawyers and the media is enough to influence the care of the dying.

All three groups step in and capitalize on the fear and confusion most people feel about death in our society. Terrified of death, desperately wanting to prolong life and wanting to end a loved one's suffering, people are profoundly confused about what to do during those last days and weeks. Embroiled in emotional and psychological dramas, people often look for cues from others as to what they should do. Unfortunately, those cues often come from lawyers, the media and extremists.

THE SAD SCIENCE OF SUSTAINING LIFE BEYOND REASON

Even without dramatic intervention, bedridden patients who are dying can live a long time if they're receiving intravenous fluids. When patients are bedridden, the demands on the various body systems (heart, lungs, kidneys, food intake) greatly diminish; with minimal care, these patients can live on for months, even in a comatose condition.

We've made tremendous advances in the technology and techniques of life support, including tubal feeding, fluid and electrolyte balance, blood transfusions, artificial respiration, electroshock, cardiac resuscitation, external and internal cardiac massage, intravenous and intracardiac injection, hyperoxygenation, blood volume and oxygen saturation measurements, anticoagulants, various surgical stomas or openings (tracheostomy, gastrostomy, thoracotomy, nephrostomy, colostomy) and dialysis. These advances make artificial maintenance of life possible almost under any condition. The original goals of these life support systems and measures was to artificially maintain life until the temporary disturbance in the functions of the body caused by accident or acute disease could be overcome. The notion was that once the patient made a recovery, these procedures could be discontinued.

Yet these procedures have been overhyped by the media to the point that everyone is aware of them and wants them to be used in every circumstance. Given the panic reaction we have to death, it was inevitable that these extraordinary procedures would become standard operating procedures. We demand that healthcare providers use every tool at their disposal to try and to reverse an irreversible process. Thus, these procedures that were originally intended for temporary management of acute and reversible conditions are now employed routinely for management of the dying process. This transition occurred insidiously, almost unnoticed, but is now complete. These modern procedures are currently used to extend the life of all dying patients for only days, weeks, or months. Never mind the tremendous cost of these modern procedures. What is reprehensible is that they are performed on people who are ill-informed about their real diagnosis and who are even given false hope of a possible cure.

To say that we're torturing patients is not an exaggeration. We put people through the worst kind of physical and mental torture before allowing them to die. It compares with the most sadistic deaths in recorded history, such as crucifixion practiced by the Romans to punish slaves, the various religious-driven tortures of the Spanish Inquisition or the pain inflicted by North American Indians on their prisoners hundreds of years ago. The stomas, experimental procedures, radical surgeries, isolation from family, silence, lies, and false promises all are the modern equivalent of driving bamboo shoots under fingernails. At least the Romans, the Spaniards, and the American Indians were honest that their goal was to torture. But the torture of dying patients is done under the guise of humanity, kindness and state-of-the-art medical care.

A side-effect of this torture is that it exacerbates our already intense fear of death. When family and friends observed a loved one's horrendous final days, weeks or months, most state they would prefer to die immediately rather than go through that prolonged and hopeless suffering. Our way of dying tremendously interferes with our way of life, even when we are in good health.

Terminal patients will call on Dr. Kevorkian rather than face the mode of death we currently impose on them. If our management of dying patients was more humane, there would be less need for such a call. Mrs. Huskins (Case #4) is an extreme example of mismanagement of a dying patient. Not all dying patients are treated that way, but most terminal patients dying in hospitals receive at least some elements of this treatment.

The Problems with Procedures

Almost any organ or system that becomes obstructed in a terminal patient is diverted through some sort of stoma. A gastrostomy is performed for a blocked esophagus; a tracheostomy for a blocked airway; a colostomy for a blocked colon; a nephrostomy for a blocked kidney; a cystostomy for a blocked bladder. Most of these blockages produce pain of varying degrees. The treating physician has the option of prescribing heavy sedation for these obstructions until death occurs (which happens quickly) or can suggest a procedure that will help the patient fight death. These procedures might provide temporary relief, but the care and maintenance of the diversion is complicated, painful, aggravating, and leads to prolonged agony or a slow death, to say the least.

When I was a physician-in-training, it was common practice to perform open chest massage on any patient with cardiac arrest. Today, with modern technology we perform closed chest massage by placing electrodes on the chest and externally stimulating the heart with a powerful electric current. Either of these two procedures can be lifesaving when presented by a patient with a sudden heart attack or drug-related cardiac arrest. But, when this occurs in a terminal patient, it is futile and even grotesque. The physician becomes a false hero, keeping the patient alive only for a few more hours or days. I am always puzzled when I observe the attitude of the family who watch the heartbeat slowly reappear on the electrocardiogram (ECG) machine, only to disappear later on. Their behavior is complex. Either they think they have witnessed the miracle of a patient brought back to life, or they are angry at the physician for not completing his miracle. In defense of the medical profession, I must add that any physician who does not perform these resuscitation procedures is exposing himself ethically and legally.

Another useless life extension procedure is the administration of intravenous fluids to terminal patients in a coma. This can extend the coma for a long time. Everyone, including the terminal patient before he lapsed into a coma, knew that death was near. What is the point of keeping patients on the brink of death for months or even years? Colleagues say You cannot let him die like that. I never understood what to die like that meant. I would ask, How can you let someone live like that?

Another futile procedure I consider useless is repeated blood transfusions. Some terminal patients can no longer form blood because their bone marrow is involved in a terminal process or because they continuously bleed through a terminally involved organ such as the stomach, kidney, uterine cervix, bowel, rectum. These patients may receive repeated blood transfusions until some other organ becomes terminally involved or until they develop a fatal blood reaction. Patients who continuously lose blood from one side of their body while continuously receiving blood on another are emotionally traumatized.

Chemotherapy is a procedure used with almost all types of cancer patients, but it is seldom used to good effect and can create tremendous pain and suffering. Physicians in charge of chemotherapy always have at hand some statistical analysis to show that any type of cancer is more responsive with chemotherapy. While it can be beneficial, it can also be a knee-jerk response to cancer. Case #8 (Robert) is a typical situation where chemotherapy was unnecessary, aggravating, and associated with complications.

These are the most frequent treatments/procedures used on terminal patients. There are many other procedures proposed by modern technology: artificial feeding is the most recent. It is a meaningful treatment for patients who have temporarily lost their ability to eat. It is unfortunately abused when forced upon terminal patients who have no interest in eating. Before implementing this procedure, the terminal patient's condition must be considered and the procedure must be fully discussed with the patient or family. Many of these procedures are used in a routine manner. Some are ordered by the medical resident or even nursing staff, as standard operating procedure. Intravenous fluids are ordered because the patient is dehydrated; blood transfusion is ordered because the patient is anemic or losing blood. A stoma is proposed because the function of the corresponding organ is blocked; dialysis is suggested because the blood accumulates toxic products, and so on. These are the answers given to patients or family, assuming they ask any questions. For instance, nobody wonders if a terminal patient in a coma is better off dying quickly of dehydration or extending life for a couple of weeks with intravenous fluids. Similarly, receiving a couple of pints of blood once or twice every week may not be appreciated by all terminal patients. What's needed is a thorough and objective analysis and discussion before each procedure is ordered; each case should be considered individually and preferences of the patient and the family should be factored into the decision.

Patients and family do not ask specific questions and doctors do not answer questions that are not specifically asked. Evasive or cautious questions get evasive or cautious answers. For instance, a nephrostomy for urinary diversion is proposed for blocked kidneys; too often the exchange of information between doctor/patient/family stops right there. Nobody discusses what is involved in dying with blocked kidneys, which could be a rapid and painless mode of death versus dying with a nephrostomy, which is painful and aggravating, and prolongs life for only a short period. If this is what the family wants, this is okay providing they know the score. Typically, people have no desire for this procedure when they know what it entails.

The Mounting Cost of Treating Dying Patients

We labor under the illusion that the more money we spend on dying patients, the more we solve the problem. Again, this illusion is allowed to take root in the absence of policies regarding appropriate financial expenditures to prolong the lives of terminal patients. The amount of money and how it is spent varies considerably depending on individual situations.

Let's start this discussion of costs with a simple truth: Keeping the terminally ill patient artificially alive with all kinds of procedures is very costly. The average rate for a bed in the emergency room or the Intensive Care Unit (ICU) is presently around $3,000 a day (though this can vary quite a bit from hospital to hospital). The strange thing, however, is that almost no one pays for it since third-party insurers pay the bill. Astonishingly, the average American incurs as much cost in medical care during the last six months of his life as during the rest of his entire life.

If the average family were asked to write a check for $30,000 for the medical care of a dying parent during the last week or two of his life, they would be outraged. Even the dying patient, given sufficient consciousness, would vigorously protest. The irony is that the average person ends up paying for this care indirectly. Third-party insurers raise the premiums to cover these costs. It's possible that this practice won't continue, since various health bills now being debated will not include coverage of terminally ill patients beyond a specified period of time. Perhaps this legislation will also shatter the myth that the more expensive the management of a dying patient is, the better it is.

Here's an example of why costs are out of control. Round-the-clock nursing care at home for a dying patient costs about $1,000.00 a day. Medicare and health insurance often covers a sizable percentage of this cost. The reason for spending this money—at least among the family of the dying patient—is that someone should be there when the loved one dies. For the family to wake one morning and find mom or dad dead is inconceivable and undesirable. No family member wants to stand guard at night, so the solution is round-the-clock visiting nurses. The fact that at least some of these nurses often are sound asleep at the moment of death doesn't seem to be a consideration.

A grandmother, rather well-to-do financially, went into a coma after a cerebral hemorrhage. She was rushed to the hospital and placed in the Intensive Care Unit ($3,000-$4,000 a day) and kept alive by all kinds of modern machines. After six months in a coma, her Medicare payments ran out and the grandmother, or rather the responsible family, was faced with this huge expense. The family transferred the patient to another center with a DNR (do not resuscitate) order, where she immediately died. This patient's cost to society was a half-million dollars, with her own assets left intact as an inheritance for the family. At present, there is no limit on the amount of money spent to keep terminally ill patients alive. The problem, of course, is that the lack of a limit presents a variety of healthcare providers with a blank check. The implicit message is: Spend as much as you need to keeping the patient alive even though you're prolonging the agony of the family rather than the life of the patient.

A man presenting with double pneumonia was brought to the hospital in a coma and with severe respiratory distress. The electro-encephalogram (EEG) showed severe, permanent brain damage. The man was placed on a respirator because he could not breathe on his own. At that moment, the family asked me for advice and I suggested that they take him off the respirator which would result in his immediate death. However, the family did not follow my advice because they received only vague answers from their own doctor. Through the use of antibiotic treatment, the double pneumonia cleared up and the patient was fully able to breathe on his own without the respirator. However, the patient was in a vegetative state and in a permanent deep coma. The family could not request that the life-sustaining procedure be stopped because he was now breathing on his own. This has been going on for two months and the patient is still alive and shows no sign of coming out of the coma.

Not only is the cost of taking care of these patients high, but it is money spent without a purpose. Because of the vague response from their doctor, they are commited to the cost of keeping someone suspended between life and death.

Doctors Don't Always Know What's Right or Best

It is a tragic aspect of human behavior that when a problem has no satisfactory answer, misleading solutions appear and multiply. Certainly we have followed the wrong path with respect to how we manage death, and doctors have been as guilty as everyone else of embracing harmful approaches. This shouldn't be surprising. As respected as physicians are today, they did not always have an illustrious history. Certain historical aspects of the practice of medicine have more in common with witchcraft than science. We forget this fact because giants of medicine such as Hippocrates (the father of medicine), Galen (Greek physician), Ambroise Pare (French surgeon), Louis Pasteur (French chemist and bacteriologist) and Albert Schweitzer (medical missionary) did so much for so many. Most of us forget that the medical profession stubbornly and ignorantly opposed Galen, Semmelweiss, and Louis Pasteur. Semmelweiss, the real father of medical hygiene, was driven to insanity by his own colleagues; he died without seeing the benefit of his discoveries. It has been argued that his premature demise was responsible for the death of thousands of pregnant women. Louis Pasteur spent most of his life challenging the scientific establishment. As recently as the previous generation, certain types of therapies used by the medical profession were shockingly backward. For instance, before penicillin and other antibiotics were discovered for the treatment of infections, pharmacology books were filled with bizarre modes of treatment that today seem barbaric. You can find decidedly unscientific recommendations for the treatment of sexually transmitted diseases (syphilis, gonorrhea) and birth control.

I point this out simply to remind you that doctors are human; they can make mistakes, they are influenced by social opinion, and they don't always speak out when their scientific knowledge should prompt them to do so. Today, many members of the medical profession have been or still are hesitant to take a firm stand on controversial issues such as abortion, birth control and AIDS treatment. It is not surprising, therefore, to see an absence of leadership by the medical profession in managing the dying patient. It is embarrassing to admit that the few regulations concerning the management of dying patients have been imposed on, rather than initiated by, the medical profession.

We cannot blame the medical profession for the lack of a cure for diseases such as cancer because our knowledge in the different sciences, such as molecular biology, is not advanced enough. When it comes to the management of dying patients, however, I consider the problems man-made or at least man-solvable. I am not saying that doctors are culpable. They do, however, have a moral and professional responsibility to take a stand on this issue. Inertia, unfortunately, seems to have the medical profession in its grip.

Though many doctors despise the current system of managing death and bitterly complain about it, they seem incapable of taking any kind of meaningful action. For instance, I recently discussed the management of dying patients with an emergency room physician. I listened to a long list of complaints this physician had, but when I noted that emergency room doctors contribute to the problem and potential solutions might hurt his income or even his career, he became defensive. Doctors as well as nurses, social workers and hospital administrators all have a vested interest in the current system, and as much as they might criticize it, they're unlikely to do what is necessary to change it.

Sometimes I even wonder if doctors extend life by a few weeks or days to allow hospitals to use the dying patient to fill up beds; to allow doctors-in-training to learn the art of survival at the expense of the dying patient; and to allow pharmaceutical companies and the equipment industry to expand their markets.

A REASON FOR CONCERN AND A CAUSE FOR HOPE

There is a good news/bad news aspect to the way we manage people's deaths today. Much of the bad news emanates from our management philosophy that says people should die in hospitals. Not only does this reduce contact between patients and families, but it creates a tense, anxiety ridden atmosphere.

I always strongly recommend that the patient return home to die within the family circle even if it means that the death comes a few days earlier than it would in the hospital. Arrangements can be made with funeral homes in advance, and the process can end in a much more peaceful, natural way. A home death is far preferable to turning hospitals into what I refer to as pre-funeral homes. Between the patient's family screaming that their mom or dad isn't receiving the proper care and the jaded attitudes of hospital staff who have seen this drama played out once too often, the final days are extremely unpleasant. Something is missing when both the dying person and his family feel that their needs are going unmet.

Typically, hospitalized patients die in a state of tremendous anxiety, confusion and isolation. Not only are they uncertain about their prognosis, they're afraid to ask anyone about it. In some instances, patients are panicked and can be driven almost mad with fear. To avoid these depths, dying people in hospitals seek refuge in denial—they delude themselves into believing they're getting better. In this hospital setting, family experience similar types of feelings, though their behaviors are a bit different—they tend to rant and rave irrationally in the face of death. Even doctors can be in denial, proposing new and ultimately futile treatments instead of facing sad realities. Other doctors deny the problem by transferring the patient to another specialist or another institution. While some doctors aren't in denial and want manage a patient's dying differently, they feel their hands are tied by laws, hospital regulations and tradition.

Despite this environment, we're also seeing some courageous healthcare professionals, patients and other groups exploring alternatives to how the process is currently managed. These aren't lone voices in the wilderness but a growing group of people who realize there has to be a better, more humane way to help people die. Though our current process of dying is ingrained in the culture, it is being challenged. Antoine de Saint-Exupéry (1950) said it in simple terms, "Il n'y a pas d'ascension sans lute contre la pesanteur —there is no ascending without fighting against gravity." No doubt, changing how we manage the death process is an uphill fight. Though there's opposition to this change, scientific and human curiosity combined with innovative ideas are slowly impacting the process.

In the middle of this fight for change are the families of those who are dying. As we'll see in the next chapter, they have a tremendous impact on the quality of the death of those they love.

CHAPTER 6

FAMILY MATTERS: FROM A HARMFUL TO A HELPFUL ROLE

Never send to ask for whom the bell tolls, it tolls for thee.
–John Donne, quoted by Ernest Hemingway

To understand the role family plays in a loved one's death, let's begin by contrasting the role family plays when animals die.

When animals' lives end, their families don't interfere in the process and are relatively (relative to humans) unaffected by it. A litter or young animals may miss their dead mothers, but it's the care rather than the presence of the mother that is missed. Animals certainly pair off in life, but the pairing is tenuous, and people tend to anthropomorphize the relationship. When an animal (such as an ape) dies in captivity, people look at the mate and say she looks sad or attribute lethargic behavior to mourning. What people do, of course, is project their own feelings on the animals or at least exaggerate what they observe. While some authors report mourning in animals (primates, elephants, lions, cats, etc.), it's not mourning of the human kind. What's observed is usually a biological bond that has been interrupted (nourishment, protection, warmth), and the infant misses the badly-needed mother. Dian Fossey (1983), for instance, reports the despair expressed by an infant gorilla after the mother was killed, and this expression of grief may seem genuine and be a mirror image of how humans express sorrow. At best, however, it is a very primitive and very temporary reflection of how we express grief.

Human death, on the other hand, is highly involving and impactful. To a greater or lesser extent, families are always an integral part of the process. From a familial perspective, it becomes a cultural or social event like a birth or a wedding, though obviously a sad rather than a happy event. The social and cultural aspects of human death shape the role families play in the process.

In Western culture, the most common and accepted emotional reaction to death is sorrow; sorrow for the dead, that is. This feeling is expressed in infinite ways by the family of the loved one. Underlying this expression is the belief that the person who has died has lost far more than anyone else through his death; that the living can somehow compensate for their loss because they are still alive.

Another cultural dictate that I've discussed earlier is that death takes places in a hospital or an emergency room. The social convention is based on the belief that only in these places can one find the scientific equipment and necessary services that might save or prolong the life of the dying person. As a result, patients approaching death always are transferred to a hospital, and emergency transfer plans are made well in advance (which ambulance company and doctor are to be called, which hospital to go to, who should go with the patient).

Third, dying at home surrounded by family is viewed as undesirable and even socially unacceptable. The social unacceptability of this notion is rooted in fears that family or friends would not know what to do should a crisis arise. People are terrified by the transition from life to death, and they would prefer to keep this horrifying episode outside of the home and confined to a hospital.

Interestingly, hospices have failed to gain widespread social acceptability; most people prefer to have their loved ones die in hospitals. Hospices don't fight death to the bitter end. Instead, their philosophical basis is an acceptance of death. Hospitals never accept death, and this willingness to fight it no matter what is much more in keeping with social norms.

Just as many families resist hospices, they also dislike euthanasia because it prematurely shortens life. Euthanasia is the response to circumstances when death is preferable to life. Many family members, however, are insulted by this response. For people who have grown up in this culture, euthanasia is selfish; it connotes an unwillingness to keep struggling, if not for one's own sake, then for loved ones.

One of the most common phrases we hear family members say is,

"At least they tried everything to keep him alive." There is an implicit cultural apology in this phrase, suggesting that we can never do enough in our fight against death. It also communicates the guilt many families feel when a loved one dies; it's as if they've been accused of contributing to the death, and they want to reassure everyone that they've done all they could. Typically, non-family members congratulate the family for all their efforts on the patient's behalf.

Within this cultural framework, the medical profession and other hospital personnel can expect to be criticized if they could have done something to prolong a life for even a few hours but didn't. Family members will routinely chastise healthcare professionals in even the most absurd circumstances if they suspect some extraordinary measure could have been instituted but wasn't. There are instances when people are brought into emergency rooms in deep comas and there's absolutely nothing that can be done for them, but families still are furious with the medical staff because they didn't try something, anything.

One of our most curious customs is to attempt to forget and replace the dead person after a period of mourning. After a decent amount of time has gone by, families talk rarely if at all about the person who has passed away. It's almost as if the person committed some unspeakable crime by dying. Whether consciously or not, families act as if the act of death was a rejection, a figurative slap in the face. People focus on replacing the person who passed away. Spouses remarry (the only way to forget the deceased), parents have another child or adopt, friends are replaced, etc. (*The Hour of Our Death*, Philippe Ariès,1982). In other words, we substitute new life to replace death, and we do so as quickly as possible. In our society, the living count for everything, the dead for nothing.

A closer examination of the mourning process demonstrates how social and cultural norms impact a family's response to death.

MOURNING

After a person dies, grief of varying intensity and duration is felt by those left behind (though for some, tremendous relief is felt instead of grief). This grief manifests itself in two ways.

In one type of grief, the mourners bemoan that the deceased person has been deprived of life. This grief is characterized by feeling sorry and sad for the departed. Implicit in this grief is the idea that the patient would have preferred life under any circumstance to death.

The other type of grief is not so much sorrow for the departed as grief driven by anger. Wives are furious because they're deprived of the presence of their husbands; sons and daughter feel like abandoned children and complain bitterly about how they've been orphaned. It is almost a selfish grief. Rather than thinking about whether the person died in peace or looked forward to death, we focus on how awful it is not to have this person here for us. This anger against the departed was well expressed by a relative of mine, who remarked about her deceased husband, "He went to rest in peace and left me alone to struggle in life."

Of course, these two types of grief are not always clearly separated in the mind of the bereaved. In general, the first type is predominant during the mourning period following death and disappears rather quickly as life goes on. The second type of grief is there from the beginning but becomes entrenched later on and time does not diminish the anger.

This is an important distinction, in that one type of grief involves an acceptance that the person they cared so much about in life is now resting peacefully, even though they still miss him. The second type has no room for this acceptance. Instead, their sorrow is derived from the dead person's absence from their lives. Persistently and stubbornly, they talk about the tragedy of someone's death, projecting their sorrow onto the person who died. For them, this person will never rest in peace.

Sorrow certainly is an appropriate and even necessary response to a loved one's death. It is a natural feeling that signifies how important and meaningful the person who passed away was to us. To feel sorrow about someone's death is a way to honor the deceased person, and not to feel sorrow would be almost an insult to their memory.

In cases of prolonged bereavement, family members often dream of the deceased. A number of people have told me that in their dreams, the person who died asked them to stop mourning for them. In other dreams, mourners create an ideal life with the departed and some have told me that they prefer their dream life to their waking life because these dreams are free of grief and sorrow.

I've also observed mourning family members who become more involved with the deceased after death than when they were alive: prayers, constant visits to the cemetery, maintenance of graves, organizing death anniversaries, pictures of the departed everywhere, keeping the house (or a specific room) as if the departed is still around and soon to come home. These people fail to understand that if their loved ones could speak, they would want only their teachings and values preserved. Anything else would be offensive and irrational. There is a time for mourning, a time for remembering, and a time for letting go. A young widow told me a dream in which her husband released her and told her to start a new life. It struck me then as now that this is exactly what these perpetual mourners need to hear. If you believe in life after death, you could make the argument that to stop mourning after a reasonable period of time is appropriate—it allows the departed to rest in peace.

In my own way, I've tried to convey this message to these mourning family members. I explain that only the living are sorry that a person has died. To maintain that the dead person would still wish to be alive is our own fear talking. If there is an existence beyond ours, who are we to conclude that the other existence is not preferable to ours? Though the process of dying is painful, we know nothing beyond that fact. When wives become professional widows or other family members become perpetual mourners, they usually are assuming knowledge that they don't possess.

When belief in heaven was widespread, priests never hesitated to insist that the departed had now joined friends and family who had previously departed, and they all were enjoying a celestial reunion. In our society where heaven no longer is a real belief for many people, the comfort of this concept is missing, prolonging the mourning period.

Family members often are involved in disagreements that revolve around someone's death. This is especially common when divorce, re-marriage and children of first and second marriages are involved. Even relatively minor issues can trigger heated conflict. Reasons for these conflicts are numerous. For instance, the son or daughter who has been taking care of a dying parent feels he and he alone should make all the decisions related to medical treatment. If anyone else dares interfere, arguments rage. Such arguments are most detrimental to the parent, who often silently watches these dramas play out and feel even more anxious and fearful because of them.

Arguments can run the gamut, from choice of doctors, decisions about medications and procedures, selection of hospitals, wills and dis-posal of assets. I have witnessed arguments about whether or not an autopsy should be performed, even before death was pronounced.

Many of these arguments stem from the family members' failures to deal with their own feelings about dying. Because tremendous fear and confusion surround their own feelings, they're unlikely to react rationally to a loved one's dying. Typically, they attempt to manage the process in odd and emotionally-heated ways, leading to all sorts of con-flicts with other family members, doctors, nurses and even the patient himself.

The clarion cry of family members is: We cannot let him die; we have to do something about it! There are three problems with this state-ment:

1. We have no power to let or not let the person die

2. We rarely ask the dying patient if we should do something about it.

3. Those who maintain that we should do something end up do-ing the wrong thing, frequently harming rather than helping the dying patient.

On the surface, these loving family members seem to have the best of intentions, but underneath they're operating out of their own fear of death. Even if the dying person is going through physical and emotional hell, the living hide their fear behind excessive and sometimes even distorted concern for the dying patient. Consciously or not, they project their own doubts, fears and uncertainties onto the dying person, making decisions for that person based on their projections rather than trying to figure out what the dying person really wants.

With this mindset, family members tend to pontificate about what's best for the dying person. They say that because someone is dying, they're not in a position to know what's best for them. To an outsider, it looks like they're not able to let go of the individual who is about to die. In reality, they're having trouble letting go of their fears of their own death.

I've observed that people have less difficulty accepting their own deaths than is commonly thought. This acceptance, however, is often thwarted by sons, daughters and other family members who consider anything less than a combative attitude to be insulting and heretical. These people should understand that the dying are often blessed with an ability to accept the end of life, and the living can help them take advantage of that ability with the proper attitudes and behaviors.

In one sense, a dying person who completely and even ecstatically embraces his death scares us to death. This person raises doubt about our values and calls into question our obsessive pursuit of pleasure. Nothing in the world is more damaging to our idea of enjoyment of life than a patient who dies peacefully and even ecstatically. It makes us wonder who is really dying and who is really living.

I have observed that some wealthy people feel rich only in relation to poor people who are crushed by their wealth. They take pleasure in depriving poor people of their dignity by flaunting their material possessions and acting as if they are superior because of what they possess. When poor people are indifferent to their wealth, however, they become insecure. Similarly, some living people need those who are dying to be terribly fearful and upset; only through the contrast of their conditions can they derive pleasure from being alive. They relish their ability to pity those who are sick and dying, and they're thrown off balance when the dying accept their own deaths or even pity the living.

Hemingway in *For Whom The Bell Tolls*, includes this famous quote from John Donne: "Never send to ask for whom the bell tolls, it tolls for thee." As the quote suggests, all of us know that death is figuratively around the corner, and this knowledge makes us reluctant to remind ourselves of this fact by talking about it. Only when death is literally around the corner are we willing to deal with our feelings about it, and that's unfortunate. Families would be able to manage the process of dying if they didn't wait until the last minute to deal with their fears and questions.

Dying people affect the living as much as the living affect the dying. There is a reciprocal exchange of information and emotions, and how each group's attitudes, words and actions have a tremendous impact on the other group's. This reciprocal exchange has received very little attention, especially in the many conferences I have attended about management of dying patients. The focus is usually on issues such as how the dying patient feels, how to relieve their pain, what to tell them and so on. I have yet to hear a doctor, nurse, family member, friend, or an acquaintance ask the following questions:

How do I feel about this impending death?

How is this death affecting me?

How does the dying patient feel about my seeing him dying?

Our Town by Thornton Wilder (1938) describes the feelings and thoughts of the dead toward the living and the indifference of the dead toward earthly matters. Interestingly, the young woman in the play who died in childbirth was irritated at her husband and the whole family for mourning her death. As rare as it is for the arts to explore this subject, it's almost as unusual to find healthcare professionals or family members exploring it.

Isolation of the Dying Patient

You would think that someone who is dying would be the center of attention; that friends and especially family would gather around and activities and conversations would include the dying person. In fact, just the opposite occurs. When family members and others hear that the condition is terminal and that someone has only so many weeks or months to live, their behavior changes. These changes can be as extreme as cutting off all contact with the person who is dying. More typical, however are the following reactions:

They lapse into periods of awkward silence when talking with the dying person.

They avoid certain subjects or words.

They repeat how much better someone is looking (whether or not it's true).

Their visits grow shorter and shorter in duration.

They avoid eye contact with the individual who is sick and appear frightened by what they perceive to be the look of death.

They appear overly concerned and are excessively caring.

All these behavioral changes effectively isolate the dying individual. Instead of feeling natural warmth and caring from family members, dying people feel as if those they care most about are acting in unnatural ways. The isolation isn't physical; it comes from the awkwardness, discomfort and fear manifested by those who the dying person loves the most.

The tragedy is that we've created this isolation relatively recently. Historically, it first appears around the time of the Renaissance (Ariès, 1992) and really took hold at the beginning of this century when fighting death became the rule and the medical profession took over management of the process. Before this, death was usually accepted and received without much struggle. The dying person was the center of human activity, the main actor in a ceremony that has completely disappeared in our modern society. Dealing with a dying patient was steeped in customs that had the strength of centuries-old tradition. Rituals were rooted in a carefully regulated ordeal for the dying and the family. These solemn procedures made death easier, and death was seen as peaceful and a relief from suffering.

The ritualistic nature of dying usually included the following steps:

1. A doctor or religious figure would inform a patient of his impending death, and then the patient would usually inform his family (rather than the doctor telling the family).

2. The dying person would confess all wrongdoing, and family members would also ask forgiveness for the wrongs they had done to the dying person.

3. The dying person would pardon those who had wronged him.

4. The dying individual would give well-considered instructions to his spouse and children and say his last goodbyes; an equitable disposition of monies and possessions would also take place; instructions for type of funeral and burial site would also be given.

The taboo that came with these rituals was: No one should do anything to delay the expected death. To do so would have been unthinkably cruel. Dying people didn't fear death. What they feared was a sudden and lonely death without this ceremony. They would have been aghast at our current practice of making this ceremony impossible by shipping people off to emergency rooms and hospitals to die.

One of the fascinating historical aspects of death is that people usually had premonitions or at least an inner awareness that they were dying (Gorer, 1965). It was assumed that the dying rather than the doctors had a better sense of their condition. Typically, someone who felt the end was near would proclaim this fact to his family with great emotion by both men and women (it wasn't until after the 17th century that men were expected to keep their emotions under control). Eventually, this emotional announcement along with the ceremonial aspects of dying began to fade away.

While we still have a ceremony today, it takes place after rather than before death. Elaborate funeral and post-funeral mourning are the norm, and they are of no comfort to the dying. Families miss the opportunity to include their loved ones in a pre-death ritual, and so the dying feel excluded from the process.

There's another reason for this isolation in our society: No one—especially not family members—talks to the dying person about how he feels about his approaching death. No one allows people to express their feelings because:

We have this false respect for the dying person's privacy and feel that asking him about his feelings would be cynical and morbid.

We're afraid to ask the question and hear the answer.

We assume that dying people aren't interested in this type of conversation because their condition turns them inward in a way outsiders can't comprehend.

Our culture frowns on this type of conversation; it is against our norms; it would signal an acceptance of rather than a fight against death.

While some dying patients are willing to discuss their feelings and family members are eager to listen and respond, most people don't have this opportunity. The tragedy of death in our present culture is its loneliness. We die alone, and our family can't share and respond to our emotions, anxieties, need for comfort and anticipation of death.

This isolation often begins during old age before any terminal disease appears. I always hear the following expression: "I want the best retirement place for my parent(s) that money can buy." The best retirement place may be a long distance away (another state or region) where family visits are limited to once a year, so the children can carry on an active social life without guilt or having their routine disturbed. Isolating parents in a condominium in another state or region is really rejection, separation from family activity and premature burial. One could make the argument that shoving an elderly person into a nearby retirement home (rather than allowing them to live in their own homes or with their family) has the same isolating impact, especially if visits are brief and perfunctory. As much as sons and daughters say they are putting parents in these homes out of love, the reality is that the consequence has the opposite effect of love. Elderly people are being cut off from everything and everyone one they know and love, and this isolation only intensifies when they're dying and transferred to a hospital.

THE FEELING OF GUILT AMONG CHILDREN

Guilt turns dying into an emotionally tortuous experience for the adult children of dying parents. Certainly dying isn't the only time people feel guilty, but it is the time when that guilt become paralyzingly intense. Children feel so guilty for their parents' deaths that it impacts their behavior not only at the time of the dying but for long afterwards. The fact that there rarely is a rational reason for this guilt is a good point at which to start a discussion of this subject.

Freud has commented extensively on guilt and relates it to the Oedipus complex (prehistoric repression of murderous feelings against the father and desire of the mother). He suggests that guilt is caused by imagined aggression that is not even carried out, insisting that fear of not controlling natural aggression is at the origin of the guilt feeling (The Ego and the Id; Sigmund Freud). Other experts in this area have connected guilt to original sin as a punishment for acquiring knowledge. What I have observed in patients who feel extreme guilt is their own irrational and excessive ego at work. When they accuse themselves of all sorts of awful behaviors toward a parent, the source of those accusations could conceivably be an overinflated ego; they believe that they and they alone are responsible for the parent's current and past suffering. My therapeutic approach is to deflate their ego and urge more humility. I also try and get them to understand that if there were to have performed all the evil deeds they feel guilty for, it would mean that they had an absurd amount of power over their parents. No one, I suggest, has that much power over another human being. Deep inside, guilt is a masochistic impulse that somehow satisfies a perverse need we have to suffer for imagined sins.

While you could probably trace the origins of guilt far into the past, it has become a defining trait of modern society. As a group we feel guilty about such issues as the ozone layer, changes in climate, pollution of rivers and oceans, tampering with world fauna and vegetation, wars, famines, epidemics and so on. We have a relatively new profession in our society—psychotherapy and social counseling—created to deal with guilt and the frustration and anger we feel when we attempt to transfer our guilt onto others.

Which brings us back to guilt and dying. The dying process activates and intensifies our feelings of guilt. Why a strong feeling of guilt is activated when parents become old, deteriorate and die is complex. The simple explanation is that children believe they could have done more for their parents when they were alive. They believe this partly because people live much longer than in the past so there are often many years for adult children to nurture and intensify their guilt. Some parents, however, are equally responsible for this situation, especially those who panic about living alone or are worried about their economic condition and manipulate their children into feeling guilty: Why don't you ever call? I'm so lonely and other familiar complaints catalyze feelings of guilt.

When parents are dying, children frequently think about or express the wish that their parents would die. Sometimes this wish emanates from a desire to see their parents not suffer any more from a disease; sometimes it's a subconscious wish because they are depressed and exhausted from taking care of a dying parent. It's not unusual for adult children to approach me and ask when their parent suffering of a terminal disease is going to die. Everyone who is burdened with the responsibility of a terminally ill patient, does, at one time or other, consider or even wish for the death of that person, even though they are providing this dying person with the best of care as well as their love. This also leads to guilt.

When guilt is omnipresent and overwhelming, it causes adult children to turn a parents' death into a nightmarish experience of blaming and anger. Two contrasting cases illustrate this point. I happened to be taking care of two patients who had terminal stages of ovarian cancer at the same time. They were in the same room and case management was more or less similar. The first patient, together with her family, was very calm and constantly praying, viewing the coming death as the will of God. The adult children had only praise for the medical care she was receiving and apologized to all the doctors and nurses for requiring their constant and diligent efforts. The second patient and her surrounding family complained bitterly. While the patient certainly was suffering, her complaints were overwhelming and often related to trivial matters. Her adult children perhaps drove her in this direction by making contradictory demands and complaining to the head nurse and hospital administrator. For instance, they insisted that a nurse and a doctor remain constantly at her bedside. When they were informed one early morning that the patient had died, they were furious that no one had told them she was about to die so they could say their last goodbyes (of course, doctors can't predict the exact moment that someone will pass away).

The first patient's children were feeling only sorrow; the second one's children were feeling mostly guilt since deep inside they blamed themselves for the coming death and found relief by transferring their guilt onto others. But, most of all, they were unable to accept death as a natural end; they were frightened of death and were looking for every possible (and even impossible) means to stop death from coming. Convinced that death is man-made, they were trying to find someone to blame for not stopping it.

Let me give you a sense of the deep level of guilt by offering you a composite portrait of how a daughter feels toward her elderly and ailing mother. The daughter believes that she can never do enough, that she does not love her mother enough. She argues with her brothers and sisters, and they accuse each other of not doing enough, and they compete in this matter. The daughter feels guilty for having outbursts of anger against her mother because her mother does not take care of herself; she feels disturbed and angry because her mother does not show interest in the care she is providing for her and constantly wonders what else she can do to improve her mother's life. The daughter is disoriented because she is now giving more attention to her mother than to her family; she is confused and depressed because deep inside she has the awful suspicion that her mother is somehow taking advantage of her (Mrs. Herman, Case #10).

This type of out-of-control guilt is rarely justified. People who willfully harm others almost never feel guilty about their actions as they easily rationalize their behavior. Caring, compassionate people are the ones most likely to feel guilty.

THE DEADLY COMBINATION: LONG LIFE AND MONEY

The combination of people living far longer than ever before and the financial issues that come with extended lives often creates great animosity between parent and child. It is no longer unusual to see people in wheelchairs, walking with canes or who are even bedridden go on living for years if proper medical and nursing care is provided.

At the same time, this extended life brings all sorts of financial issues into play. There's a tremendous fear of being incapacitated, which prompts more than one person to arrange for round-the-clock nursing care if they become an invalid. Other elderly people take out all sorts of insurance in response to their fear of being alone and abandoned. Many people do estate planning with a provision that money be set aside for terminal care.

Many of these issues were a moot point until relatively recently. It used to be that adult children provided care for parents until the end, taking them into their homes and nursing them in the best way they could. This is now much more the exception than the rule. As a result, elderly people often panic as they contemplate the end of their lives; they resent their children (when they were younger, they may have provided their dying parents the care their children won't provide) who consider this care someone else's responsibility.

Given this environment, all sorts of tension-producing decisions are inevitable. I've seen many senior citizens determined to spend as much as they can before they die. Others reserve much of their money for what they anticipate will be enormous healthcare and retirement costs. Some adult children resent how their parents are using this money, believing that they're out of their minds or paranoid about the future. Some children even take legal action to protect their inheritances, but they are usually unsuccessful unless they can prove complete irresponsibility on the part of their parents. Whether it's legal action or simply heated arguments between parents and children, these issues often hurt or even destroy loving relationships.

When people are dying, these problems intensify. When we die, we have to give up our wealth and power, and dying people cling desperately to these things. To be rich and accumulate wealth has become a kind of cult in our society, almost a necessity in our free enterprise system where jobs, education, health coverage and retirement are not fully guaranteed. The result is that every human being has to create savings and wealth during his adult life to secure a good living and medical care after retirement. The consequences of creating these savings can get out of hand, and there is no limit as to how much wealth is accumulated. Becoming rich is no longer a means to an end, but the end itself. This is tragic for dying people. Life becomes money and money becomes life, but at the time of dying one has to surrender wealth the way one has to surrender everything else.

Some of these wealthy people hold onto their fortunes as if it were life itself. They have great trouble parting with their money, of passing it on to future generations. Any conversation with their children about who gets what is bound to explode into recrimination. Some of these people have great difficulty making out a will or making one out that gives their children a reasonable inheritance.

The Evil Death

Avenge yourself, become a problem for your children in your old age, is a popular quotation. Some elderly people become nasty as they're dying. While the dying process can and should bring out the best in us, it often brings out the worst. I've seen people who have led positive, good lives changed by their impending death.

To understand how the dying process changes a constructive life to a destructive one, we need to look at libido and destruction. These two concepts are motivations for living. Libido dominates in youth and adulthood, and while destruction may be present during a whole lifetime, it may dominate in old age. Usually when a person is active in adulthood, the tendency is libidinal (constructive), but when one retires and becomes idle, there is a tendency to become selfish, demanding and destructive. A relationship between a retired or inactive person and the surrounding people (often his children) can become destructive. The old spinster in <u>La Terre</u> by Emile Zola is typical of this destructive personality.

When this destructive personality emerges, it results in what I refer to as an evil death. The dying person is fully aware of his impending death and has been secretly or openly hateful to surrounding family and friends. What this person resents most is that after his departure life will still go on. Not only does he resent being absent from the world, but he would like to see the world completely disappear at the time of his death. If his life has to end, he does not want to die alone. Adolf Hitler, who wanted Germany and even the whole world to disappear with him, is an extreme example of this attitude. Without going to this extreme, some people try to make their dying as uncomfortable as possible for their adult children. They do this in a variety of ways, though making their children feel guilty is probably the most common. They demand to be the center of attention and make others feel they're being selfish if their attention wanders. Using the threat of disinheritance as a weapon, they derive a perverse enjoyment in making their kids squirm. It should come as no surprise that these people's deaths are a relief to everyone.

RESTRUCTURING THE RELATIONSHIP

Underlying all the issues discussed in this chapter is the need for a fundamental shift in the relationship between parents and their children. This shift is necessary because of two relatively new (historically speaking) trends:

Families are smaller. It's not unusual for one or two children to bear the burden of caring for an aging, debilitated and dying parent. While three, four or more children could spread out the responsibilities in the past, today one adult child is often the only one available for these duties (sometimes because our mobile society has seen other siblings move to other states or countries).

Aging parents live longer. Not only do they live longer, but they're more debilitated, require more expensive care and hang on for months or even years when they're severely ill or incapacitated.

When these elderly people are dependent on their adult children, terrible tensions and resentment surface. These adult children don't have the resources—financial as well as emotional—to make the traditional relationship work. The role reversal of aging parents becoming dependent on their children is demeaning to both parties. What we need to do is redefine what it means to be an older adult, to carve out a place for these people in our society so that they're independent and empowered to make their own decisions. The relationship between the elderly and their adult children should be equal and interdependent. If we could set up this type of relationship, much of the guilt and anger that surfaces when adult children care for dying parents would be eliminated. If parents retained their dignity and their freedom to choose what they feel is best for them—and if they didn't feel beholden to their children—the last few months and years of their lives would be more meaningful and peaceful.

Chapter 7

HOW THE ELDERLY REALLY FEEL
ABOUT DYING AND DEATH

Il ne faut pas avoir peur de la mort, c'est une douce amie—One should not be scared of death, it is a sweet friend. –Montaigne

Persistent Memories

As opposed to past generations that believed they would go to heaven or hell after dying, most people today believe only life exists and that our body and soul disappear after we lose that life (Ariès, 1982). As a result of this view, we look at our approaching deaths and see nothing but doubt, pessimism and fear. The only salvation for many of us is how we're remembered by those we leave behind either the family, or friends, or any circle we lived in. I refer to this concept as persistent memory, and as we'll see, it often exacerbates tensions between adult children and their dying parents.

Belief in persistent memory barely existed during the Middle Ages or even before. At a time of literal Christianity, people were not concerned with the legacy they left on earth but solely with how to prepare oneself for Heaven. Limited attention was paid to proper distribution of inheritance but significant contributions were made to the church as a way to pay for a seat in Heaven. In the year 1000, which was expected to be the end of the world, the Church was richer than ever because of immense donations. Dying people were paying handsomely to be buried within the Church or at least in the immediate vicinity. No attention was paid to the world left behind except for epitaphs on the tombs inviting passersby to pray for the souls of the dead. In fact, dying people wrote wills stipulating that heirs must pray for their souls.

As atheism spread and belief in an afterlife waned, people embraced persistent memory. In fact, it became a significant catalyst to the formation of families (because children and their grandchildren are the best and most likely candidates to keep that memory alive). Dying parents often express the wish that their children remain united. What they mean by this—though it may not be explicitly stated—is that they want them united around the memory of the parent (or parents). A grave easily and frequently visited by family and friends is the dream of people dying today.

The fear is that we will be quickly forgotten; we wish to remain a memory for as long as possible. What counts now is not so much whether we go to Heaven or Hell but what we accomplished in life and how it is remembered after death. The quality and the duration of the memory we're going to leave behind becomes increasingly important as death draws near. It represents our best chance of reaching some kind of afterlife when we die. We stay alive for as long as the people we left behind remember us. Although this type of life after death exists for only a relatively small number of years after we die, it satisfies almost everyone because we will remain a part of our family, our circle of friends and others after death. Before we die, we derive great satisfaction from imagining our children saying, "If Mom or Pop were alive, they would have done it this way." This is the modern version of heaven.

The problem with this focus on persistent memory is that it adds to our fear as death approaches. Dying parents fear that their children will soon forget them as their grief passes and their lives return to normal. Parents are also scared that their children won't remember them fondly; that their memories will be inaccurate at best and negative at worst. The subject lies unspoken between them, too emotional and complicated to be brought into the open.

An alternative to persistent memory is to fulfill one's mission or purpose while on earth and leave that not only to family but to everyone. It doesn't matter what that purpose is, whether it's of the Nobel Prize type or is quite mundane. The only thing that's important is that they feel that they were put on earth to accomplish a given mission, and once it's completed, it's perfectly natural to die. It doesn't matter if statues are erected in your honor or even if your family believes you're the most brilliant, brightest, kindest person who ever lived. Receiving credit isn't the point. What's important is that you did what you did. There is a Japanese film, Ikiru, by Kurosawa. In this film, Ikiru struggled to open a neighborhood park before he died. He didn't care about being given credit. What mattered to him was the park he wanted to build and nothing else. Others took credit, but he did not care.

Orthodox Judaism adheres to the following definition of life after death: "It is made of the memory you leave after you departed, the persistent effect of your actions while you were alive, and the continuous influence on the living even after you die." You do not have to be remembered as an individual but the persistent effect you leave after you are gone defines your existence after death. Orthodox Jews do not deny a real existence of Heaven and Hell, but they are vague about it and consider it of limited importance.

Today, dying people find comfort in the knowledge that we did what we were supposed to do while we were alive. By fulfilling our purpose, we impacted many people in countless ways. Persistent memory is concept that has become embedded in our culture. The world of art gives us ample evidence of this fact. The poem, "Eulogy Written in a Country Churchyard" by Thomas Gray, and the painting, *Persistence of Memory* by Salvador Dali are just two examples.

Old age in the second half of the 20th century is different than old age in previous centuries. Without the advantages of modern medicine and improved living conditions, people were more accepting of death because it provided relief from a very difficult life. A common prayer for the dead went: The load was getting heavy and God closed his/her weary eyes." A spiritual referred to death as freedom at last.

Today, life has been extended and improved to the point that it's difficult to let go and say, enough. Though we all possess a natural instinct that prompts us to accept death as our life draws to a close, that instinct has been circumvented by a variety of factors unique to this era.

Let's look at those factors and how they contribute to the increasing difficulty we have not only with death but with the second half of our lives.

A Dark Cloud

We live under, and are continuously influenced by, the shadow of death. Indeed, our philosophy of death has become our philosophy of life; we are no longer living but are constantly dying. To some this may seem an overstatement, especially to younger people who are engaged in all sorts of meaningful activities. In fact, the very intensity of our adult life can often be a way to shield ourselves from our fear of dying. We become workaholics to ward off stagnation (which suggests a death-like state) and fill every second of our leisure time with activities to prove to ourselves that we are alive. As long as we're working and physically vigorous, this frenzied activity is effective. As soon as we slow down—when we retire or when we no longer possess the energy or ability to be so active—then the fear of death hits us hard.

Given the scientific and economic progress we've made, old age should be a tremendously rewarding and satisfying part of life. Having achieved financial security, developed hobbies and interests and ful-filled family commitments, we should enjoy the freedom and satisfac-tion these golden years offer us. Too often, however, these last years are fool's gold. Our preoccupation with and way of managing death turns old age into a terribly difficult time. We observe how others die, and it's frightening. We see friends and relatives in wheelchairs, on life support systems, suffering in hospitals and devastated by anxiety and depression.

When we know our time is getting near, the obsession with dying can take on a nightmarish aspect. Some people think of nothing but when, where, and how they are going to die and whether or not some-one will be present when they are dying. In others, this state of mind takes on such hysterical proportions that they no longer know if they fear death or if they wish to die. Some may even wish they were never born (irrationally believing that the agony of dying and death makes life not worth living), and many feel that the price of extending life is not worth the accompanying mental and physical suffering. They with-draw, and it is difficult to know if they belong to the world of the living or the dead. More than one person has told me they feel like a prisoner on death row.

What's interesting is that a significant number of people have rebelled against this attitude. Despite the societal terror of dying, absurdly extended lives and the medical mismanaging of the process, some people have found a different way to approach old age.

A Healthier Approach to the Last Part of Life

I've had friends and patients who chose not to fight against but ignore old age. To give you some insight into this mindset, here is how this type of person might express his philosophy:

I love life so much! To be crippled, in a wheelchair, in need of constant nursing care, a nuisance to my family, others, and even myself, is not really living. It is an insult to life. I love life too much to settle for anything but being productive, active, useful to myself, family, and others. I would not want to be a pitiable spectacle or recipient of inadequate care. I want to be remembered as vital, as the envy of those who knew of me and of my accomplishments. To sully my accomplishments by spending months or years in an unproductive and dependent state is not something I want. I also do not want any self pity; it is not the picture I want to leave behind.

People who have been leaders, achievers and doers for most of their lives want to die at their desks or on the job. They are kings of their worlds, and they cannot tolerate the thought of their enemies seeing them handicapped or impotent. Their pride in who they are and what they've done supersedes and shuts down most of the fear; they want to die as they lived—if not in battle, then at least not in shame and helplessness.

It's important to note that many of these people have become more productive and creative in the years after middle age, and that this is against all the laws of nature. Until recently, this was never possible. The elderly may have been respected in certain cultures, but they were considered useless when it came to work, parenting and other tasks. The great myth many people labor under is that we become less productive and creative as we age. More often than not, creativity blossoms in old age. Many artists (Picasso, Eugene Ormandy, Robert Frost) and great scientists and philosophers (Albert Einstein, Charles Darwin, Martin Buber) have been creative past middle age.

The myth persists despite our transition from physical to intellectual labor. When work was measured by fields plowed and bridges built, it made some sense to view the second half of life as far less productive. But humans are the only species where mental output is more important than physical output. Octogenarians can remain vigorous mentally, These people—especially if they're creative—tend to die at a ripe old age and while still working. One of the keys for these creative, productive senior citizens is that they don't doubt the value of their work. Unlike other elderly people who feel useless, these individuals are buoyed by their contributions to organizations and society. They die with their boots on and refuse to spend their last years fretting about their approaching deaths.

The Courageous Elderly:
A Trend Toward Looking Death Squarely in the Eye

While a less religious society fears death more than in the past, a less religious society also makes it easier to accept death. This paradox has to do with the concept of judgment day. While the reward of heaven might make someone embrace death, the punishment of hell might make one terrified of that final moment and what comes next. As people have become less and less religious, they no longer are driven by the terror that they'll go to hell.

Without that terror of punishment, there is room to look at death differently. Suddenly, it is its own reward. Non-existence may appear attractive to those who are mentally, physically and spiritually spent. They are tired of life and ready to rest. As frightening as it might appear to some, a permanent sleep with total unconsciousness is welcome by others. With the threat of eternal damnation removed, people have changed their ideas about what death means. In one sense, this new attitude is a reaction against the clergy. Not having to account for every action performed during a lifetime is a blessed relief for some. Religious leaders are well aware of the negative impact of their fire and brimstone sermons, and many of them have softened their stances—even religion has taken some of the sting out of death. While certain rituals are still performed and lip service is given to the concepts of heaven and hell, they don't hold the same power as they once did.

Out of all this comes a revelatory notion: Death is not as frightening to dying people as everyone assumes it is. If this seems like a contradiction to my earlier statements that people approach death and dying with terrible anxiety and fear, bear with me a moment. My thesis is that among the people I've been discussing in this chapter—the productive, the creative, the ones who don't believe in eternal damnation—there is far less fear than we might imagine. It's not as hard for them to face the fact that they're going to die as we might believe.

If we only look intellectually or objectively at those who are dying, we'll jump to the wrong conclusion. When someone accepts death, he is doing so not just with his mind, but with his emotions and spirit as well. As much as his mind might harbor doubts and fears about death, his spirit is ready for its approach. Consciously or not, elderly people are starting to discover that extended life has been stretched to the limits of how long they wish to live. There is a time when one has had enough of earthly life: to wake up every morning and go to sleep every evening, to be exposed to weather variations, to feel innumerable aches and pains, to worry about money (whether rich or poor), to feel isolated and lonely. The list of things we've had enough of is long. This is the time when we wish to die.

At an advanced age, some people slowly start to withdraw from the world of the living and move slowly toward the world of the dead and an abstract existence after death (Tibetan Book of the Dead, Evans-Wentz, 1960). They recognize that there is nothing wrong in non-existence after death, are not afraid of it and even are attracted to it. They slowly and progressively realize that the values of the living may be trivial or meaningless and lose interest in many of the things they were attached to when they were younger (money, family, friends, etc.).

They withdraw to a special world. The extrovert becomes an introvert (as described in Jungian psychology) and no longer values a social life. These individuals are really preparing themselves for a new world or no world at all. They are obsessed with but not afraid of death. They are not always understood by the living and even may be called senile. The truth is that some of these elderly people no longer belong to the world of the living; they already have stepped into the world of the dead and are very much at ease with it. To the surrounding family, this is a shock. That any one would lose interest in life and desire to stop living seems incomprehensible. Many younger people resent and are angered by old people (mostly old parents) wishing to die.

For me, it is a constant and hopeless struggle to convince family members that terminally ill, 85-year-old Mom or Dad does not need a surgical procedure or a new miracle treatment. The sad part is that these new procedures sometimes are proposed and promoted by the medical profession, specifically by the new generation of specialists who always have at hand a new protocol of treatment for any kind of terminal disease. When astute sons and daughters ask probing questions about the treatment before signing the consent form, the treatment is rarely performed. The answers to those questions dissuade most adult children from extending their loved one's life even one more day, given the discomfort and pain and generally poor quality of life that will ensue.

Though dying parents can't always articulate their feelings on these matters, my sense is that they're usually in agreement with their children when the decision is made not to extend life. It takes tremendous courage, maturity and a great amount of love on the part of the children to let their parents go when they have reached this stage. Unfortunately, many adult children can't let go. Too often, I've witnessed these sons and daughters forcing their parents to undergo all kinds of painful and futile medical or surgical procedures.

If you could see into the heart and soul of people who are dying, you would see two opposite desires at work. One desire is to hold on to life because they're afraid of separating from the surrounding universe. The other desire is to leave because they feel detached from and are no longer participating in the surrounding universe. It might come as a surprise to many that the latter desire often holds sway.

At times during my career, I have informed patients that they were soon to die. In most instances, the patients remained calm and even smiled, saying they knew it all along, but the surrounding people who heard the death sentence reacted with horror and panic. It is often because of this reaction that many elderly parents keep on living, fearing that their wish to die may be resented and considered an insult by their children. In other words, they choose to live a miserable few more months to please their children.

What Elderly People Know that Younger People Don't

Some authors have revealed a strange truth about extended life and death in old age. What's strange is their implications that healthy people surrounding the dying should be in charge of the process and how they should die.

In "Living Too Long" (New York Times Magazine, January 14, 1996), Harvey R. Moody of Brookdale Center on Aging at Hunter College in New York, states that old age is too much dependency on others; George L. Maddox, Director of the Long-Term Care Research Program at Duke University, says that people in old age are too dependent with no promise, no hope, no redemption; Erickson (1950) concludes that we let old people struggle against their failing biology, and we expect too much from them.

Letting Go: A Hospice Journey (produced by Susan Froemke and Douglas Graves, edited by Deborah Dickson and Albert Maysles; HBO, New York), proposes a team of professionals to assist in the last moments of dying.

Many philosophers and healthcare observers have reached the conclusion that elderly people should be told how and even why they are to die; that older people naturally become dependent at this stage in their lives and that it makes sense that younger, healthier people take over the decision-making process as these people are dying.

In reality, the trend I've observed is the opposite of what these authors are saying. Elderly people are demanding more of a say in the way they die and less interference from family and healthcare professionals. Certainly it's still very common for people to interfere in and take over decision-making from the elderly. Things will really change only when the fear of death diminishes, economic independence from surrounding family is established and as senior citizens organize themselves and lobby for their rights.

Having witnessed the difficult deaths of contemporaries, a growing number of older people are asking questions, expressing opinions, and even making decisions: about the mode of treatment when terminally ill, signing a DNR order (do not resuscitate), living wills, cremations, funeral arrangements, type of burial, and so on. While this is done with some hesitancy on the part of the dying and occasional opposition on the part of the family, this independence movement is growing.

I don't want to make it sound as if elderly people who are dying are uniformly able to make rational decisions in the final months, weeks and days of their lives. This is a subject dominated more by irrationality than rationality, more by emotion than intellect, more by anger and guilt than acceptance and more by fear than courage. For these reasons, I never mention this subject to senior citizens unless they mention it first. Still, they are mentioning it first more and more often. When they start talking about these issues, I usually limit myself to the observation that we do not know and as yet have not found out how to die in old age. I also stress that the older we get, the more incapacitated we become and the more painful it is to die. To those willing to continue the conversation and when the circumstances are favorable, I often ask, "Do you sometimes think of death?" and "Assuming you have a choice, how would you like to die?"

People's responses to these questions have demonstrated that old people are preoccupied with death, that they constantly fear/wish for death and they do not know how to approach it. Whenever possible, I tell them what I believe: that old age can be a beautiful experience and it has the potential to be the most significant part of life *if and only if* the fear of death can be addressed.

In any discussion of how we die, there are ironies, and one of these ironies is that we're extending life negatively. Though we have the means to help people live longer than ever before, it's often not worth the effort; the longer we live, the more suffering we're forced to endure. At first blush, it seems that the people who live the longest have the best lives. In fact, the people who live the longest are subject to the most physical and emotional pain.

Part of the problem is that younger people don't always know what older people do. While both fear death, younger people don't realize that when you age, you become ready to die; you begin to accept and even look forward to the peace that comes with death. Instead, they look at death as this horrifying abyss that they want to prevent everyone from falling into. Given this fear, they have institutionalized the life-at-any-cost philosophy; they advocate keeping people alive no matter the price financially or in suffering. Ultimately, it will result in a society burdened with too many old and debilitated people. If our approach to dying doesn't change, this burden will be difficult for future generations to bear.

A DELICATE BALANCE

We reach a point where our desire to live is counterbalanced by our desire to die. Usually we reach this point later in life, when we start to fail emotionally and physically. As this failure progresses, the balance shifts in favor of the desire to die. As strong as our survival instinct might be, it is not strong enough to keep the two desires in balance.

Previous generations reach this point much sooner than we do today; medical and social progress has not only extended life but the quality of life. While it once was normal to die between ages 50 and 60, today it is normal to live and to live better than ever before. Still, at some point the desire to die gains more weight. Usually this is a gradual process followed by a precipitous decline. Something goes terribly wrong with our minds or bodies, and science can do little to stop the decline. It's not simply that we're getting less joy out of life; we can tolerate the gradual diminishment of pleasure, satisfaction and challenge. What we can't tolerate is the loss of joy and meaning; this tips the scales in favor of a desire for death. We are left with only a shadow of our former life, and when this shadow is sustained artificially by medical technology, our minds find it horrifying. Unfortunately, our desire to die is buried deep within us. We don't bring it to the surface because societal norms forbid it. As much as we might wish for a peaceful death, we can't articulate it for fear of disappointing our doctors and saddening our children.

What everyone needs to realize is that most people, if allowed to express their true feelings, would wish to end their lives when fully informed about their terminal conditions. In fact, some of these people might even request doctors to hasten their departure. To believe otherwise is a pipedream. Elderly people understand the desire to die far better than younger, healthy individuals.

Dying Patients' Rights

Families need to put themselves in the place of those who are dying and attempt to see the world through their eyes. Perhaps if they did, they would not be so quick to exploit the dying. While much has been written about the American way of death and how the grief of mourners is exploited for commercial gain, the larger issue of exploitation revolves around those who are in the process of dying but not dead yet. In a sense, the living exploit the dying in order to find out what death is like. There's a morbid fascination with the process, and just as we slow down to gawk at the scene of a car accident, so too do we scrutinize our loved ones who have only weeks left to live. We treat them like accident victims rather than as we have always treated them—as people who need and deserve our love. We become too much observers of their dying rather than caring participants.

Since people who are dying are weak and vulnerable, we can also easily overpower them and treat them as we wish. Many times, I've seen family members treat their usually older parents or grandparents as if they were helpless children. They take away their decision-making power and rob them of their dignity. All this makes the dying even more afraid than they already are, and they are so scared that they do what people tell them.

Just because someone has a terminal illness doesn't mean they've lost their ability to reason and feel. In most cases, only their bodies are affected by disease. Though drugs may cause them to be disoriented, most dying people are perfectly capable of making rational decisions. Unfortunately, we—families, doctors, friends—tend to make their decisions for them. It strikes me that a Dying Patient's Bill of Rights would be helpful, and not just from a legal sense. It would serve notice to families that the people they care about have not been reduced to the status of children or brain-damaged adults because they don't have long to live.

I often wish that sons, daughters and other relatives of dying patients could hear what their loved ones are thinking about them. If they could, this is what many of them would hear:

I would not mind dying if my kids would just leave me alone.

I don't want to be burdened with my family's fear, repulsion of death and false sympathy.

I don't like the way my brothers and sisters pull away from me because I'm dying and blame me for the absence my death will produce.

I wish my family would just be themselves and let me die in my own way.

If family members knew how the dying person is seeing them, feeling about them and judging them, they might change the way they act.

Chapter 8

DOCTORS AND HOSPITALS:
DIVINITY, BUREAUCRACY AND OTHER ILLS

"I changed his dressing, and God cured him" –Ambroise Paré

To understand the present role doctors play in treating dying patients, we need to look to the past. The way doctors view dying patients and the way dying patients and their family and friends view doctors has been shaped by events that occurred thousands of years ago. Before exploring the current impact, we need to go back in time and understand the origins of attitudes toward and harbored by physicians.

SUPERNATURAL POWERS, SCIENTIFIC REALITIES

As consciousness was rising in prehumans and primitive men and women, the need to understand the universe also was rising. The earliest explanations were simple magic: Supernatural entities were governing the universe and making things happen. Once people acknowledged and accepted these magical forms, the next problem was how to communicate with and influence them. Primitive people convinced themselves that there must be some technique, language, or ritual that would allow them to communicate with supernatural authorities. Sorcerers and witches were anointed to talk to and influence these divinities. These sorcerers never presented themselves as magical, but rather as intermediaries between the common people and the divinities; the divinities alone determined whether to grant people's requests. This intermediary role protected shamans from verbal and physical abuse in case the request was not granted.

Typically, requests were for a cure for disease or to spare the life of someone dying. Even when shamans prescribed medications (mostly herbs), they did so with the understanding that the herb had some magical power transmitted from the divinities.

The separation of magic from rational medicine based on scientific knowledge started with the ancient Greeks. Aristotle and Hippocrates practiced rational medicine in the same era where priests and priestesses transmitted requests for a cure from the sick to the Gods in the Temple of Aesculapius. The separation of cure through magic or by priests from medical cure by doctors has characterized the Occidental civilization starting with the Greeks, while the rest of the world remained focused on magic or spiritual cures.

Belief in a supernatural power is almost innate in humans, and it's logical to speculate that this belief started in prehistory with the rise of consciousness. During this time, shamans were the only ones who administered medical care. Though shamans, witch doctors and wizards have largely disappeared from our culture and doctors with science-based medicine have taken their place, it would be a mistake to dismiss this ancient form of healing. Whether consciously or not, many people still believe in the magical power of non-medical remedies. The current trend toward mind-body healing, the way certain evangelical religious groups subscribe to the laying on of hands as a cure for all sorts of diseases and the use of everything from hypnosis to prayer to deal with serious physical problems harkens back to shamanistic healing. It might not be a conscious process, but many sick and dying people don't separate scientific treatment from an alternative, non-scientific approach. At the same time that they're receiving treatment with state-of-the-art technology, they're praying for divine intervention or practicing guided imagery therapy. As an obstetrician attending births of people around the world, I've been amazed by the variety of taboos and rituals that are part of the process (even among highly educated, affluent people).

Given all this, it should not be surprising that over time, the supernatural powers that once belonged to shamans have been transferred to physicians.

THE DANGER OF DOCTORS PLAYING GOD
(OR OF PATIENTS PERCEIVING THEM THIS WAY)

As atheism spread and religious dogma began to be interpreted figuratively rather than literally—and as medicine advanced and doctors were looked upon as miracle workers—they assumed a more powerful role in people's minds. To someone without strong religious convictions and who lacked scientific knowledge, doctors appeared to possess divine healing powers. Some doctors accepted and even embraced this divine aura.

To a certain extent, this god-like mystique benefits patients. It gives them great confidence in their physicians, and this confidence may make treatment more effective. Because medicine is both an art and a science—and because there is much science can't explain about how medicine works—an almost religious faith in one's doctor may not be a bad thing in certain circumstances.

Most doctors, however, shy away from this role of miracle worker and have learned to separate their scientific knowledge from their curative powers. This separation is aptly symbolized by Ambroise Paré, a physician in the French Army during the Renaissance, who was famous for his skill in healing wounds by keeping them clean. He essentially said, "I changed his dressing and God cured him." In a way, he was a precursor of Semmelweiss and Pasteur.

The modern doctor combines the science and art of medicine. As scientist, he relies on a body of knowledge and applies it in his diagnosis and treatment. As artist , he walks a fine line between intuition and the old belief in magic and supernatural power. The danger is when doctors cross this line or when patients perceive that they're capable of doing so. There are doctors who can sense something is wrong or who intuitively know what their x-rays or other pieces of technology don't tell them. Much of this educated guess-work is a result of extensive experience, and it should not be portrayed as magical. Still, the art of medicine often suggests to patients an uncanny, almost god-like ability to treat and cure.

THE MIRACLE WORKER

When patients are dying, society's ambiguous perspective on doctors often emerges in dramatic and instructive ways. Let's take a moment and examine why this perspective is ambiguous.

On the one hand, the public praises modern medicine for all the progress it has made in extending and improving people's lives. Many of us now live into our eighties with a good quality of life. The news media constantly reports impressive lifespan statistics as well as reports on all types of medical breakthroughs. In reality, doctors should not be receiving most of the credit for the discoveries reporters give them. Many times, biologists, pharmacologists, chemists, physicists and others in the scientific community are responsible for these initial advances. The medical profession, however, tests and delivers them to the public. As the go-between, doctors attract the lion's share of both blame and credit when these new treatments fail and succeed.

While most people intellectually understand that doctors are human and can't work miracles, their emotions thwart that understanding. Emotionally, people often believe they should live forever in excellent health, and that when they (or a loved one) becomes sick and are dying, then the fault lies with doctors. Why, they wonder, didn't they exercise their special healing powers; there must be something in that black bag that will work. On many occasions, I've seen doctors blamed when:

A woman gives birth to a child with a congenital malformation.

A man, who is declared in good health by his doctor the week before, suffers a heart attack.

A malignancy develops a year after a patient has been declared free of disease.

I remember once during a patient's yearly check-up, I found a very early cancer of the ovary. It would have been very easy to miss, and I was lucky that I discovered it. Expecting praise for detecting this problem early, I was surprised to hear the patient's family grill me about why I didn't spot the problem a year earlier. I cite this example not to criticize patients and their families but to demonstrate how easy it is to expect miracles from doctors at times of emotional stress.

More Open-Minded and Less Omnipotent Doctors

Interestingly, doctors have the same type of ambiguous feelings about themselves that the public has. We are bound by the Hippocratic Oath to heal and extend a useful and happy life (and those who violate this Oath through incompetent or unethical actions are usually censored or lose their license to practice). At the same time, however, doctors aren't always sure how to go about fulfilling this Oath though we act as if we're sure. In other words, we feel we should know what to do but don't always have the answers. In a society that views doctors as miracle workers, this is a difficult admission to make.

I will never forget the advice given to me by one of my former teachers when I was a resident-in-training. He used to say that the best answer a physician could give to any question is, "I do not know." To the angry retort: "You are a doctor, you should know," the humble reply should be, "What doctors know about the human body is limited."

There is a difference between the Holy Bible, which is presented as a divine inspiration with an answer for everything, and medical textbooks, which summarize human medical knowledge but is incomplete, filled with uncertainties and errors and in need of constant revisions and additions. No textbook author is an absolute authority. Doctors themselves, unfortunately, often contribute to the false impression that medicine has an answer for any malfunction of the human body. On occasion, doctors feel obliged to hide their ignorance behind Latin, Greek or scientific jargon that may describe the problem but does not explain anything.

Doctors who refuse to admit they don't know often believe that only medical care administered by bona fide professionals can cure diseases. Any non-medical or even spontaneous cure is ignored or considered doubtful. Most members of the medical profession refuse to acknowledge the fact that many cures are non-medical in origin or at least outside the realm of classic medicine.

Physicians have a specific term, placebo effect, for this kind of cure, which is why they use placebo drugs. From the medical point of view, placebo means that an ineffective medication was administered to a sick patient who believed that the medication would be effective and so was cured anyway. Sometimes a patient follows an alternative treatment at the suggestion of some friends (such as herbal medicine, for instance) and it works.

What's difficult for doctors to remember—and the reason that many patients are intimidated into silence about alternative approaches—is that many cures are spontaneous, that the body has the potential to heal itself (close its own wounds, fight infections, etc.) and that all modes of treatments are not known to the medical profession. When people are dying, they are susceptible to anything that offers hope. Many times, they mix both medical and non-medical medicines and treatments. Lately, non-medical methods of healing have gained public recognition and are even subjected to scientific investigation (statistical analysis, control series, etc.). The most popular as of this writing are chiropractic, acupuncture, naturopathy, and homeopathy.

When I am asked for my advice about a non-medical treatment that interests a patient, I always encourage it if I am convinced it's not harmful; I know they will try it anyway. I try to relieve their embarrassment because their optimism about a given pill or treatment approach increases the odds of it being effective.

Fake Medicine

People who are dying (or their families) are more likely to believe in magic than other patients. They desperately want something to work, and they are open to all possibilities. This makes them likely targets for snake oil salesmen. Fake medicine is the conscious abuse and deception of a gullible patient. The line between fake medicine and legitimate alternatives, however, is not always clear. Doctors need to be alert to the former and open to the latter.

It is easy to take advantage of panic in the dying patient and family. I was once asked to join a committee for the purpose of giving support and comfort to patients with advanced cancer. I eagerly accepted, hoping to learn more about this type of patient. What I subsequently learned was frightening. The committee was headed by two rather aggressive women who repeatedly mentioned that they both had advanced cancer

(Stages III and IV), that they were given only a few months to live, and that now (thirteen and seven years later, respectively) they were alive and well. Their purpose, they said, was to make available to all people with advanced cancer the mode of therapy that had been so effective for them. They also wanted open debate on the different modes of cancer treatment so that the patients could be properly educated.

In one sense, all this is fine and I routinely provide my patients and their families with information about all the alternatives available. Still, doctors need to be vigilant. For instance, I was informed that this committee was sponsored by a group of doctors who specialized in chemotherapy and who were subsidized by a drug company. At that point, I questioned the real motivations of this committee.

Was this legitimate or fake medicine? Certainly I had my suspicions. It's also easy to dismiss what seems fake and is actually tremendously effective. Not so long ago, most doctors would have laughed about the medicinal benefits of aspirin, red wine and green tea.

There has been a great deal of debate about the efficacy of many standard treatment procedures. Cancer chemotherapy, for instance, is often misunderstood and attacked. It is a very difficult field of medicine. A complete cure is rare from chemotherapy, and many of these complete cures would have occurred anyway since they are associated with surgery and/or radiotherapy, which are the real curative measures. Chemotherapy is only an adjuvant and precautionary measure. What chemotherapy often does is extend life before recurrence of disease, and most of all it extends the quality of that remaining life because the patient returns to normal activity during that period of relief. Therefore, chemotherapy is not fake medicine but a misunderstood branch.

To have this debate transferred from the privacy of the doctor's office to an assembly composed of individuals with advanced cancer could be a horror. During my career I have attended many conferences given by healers and miracle workers. Audiences are gullible—they want to believe if they or loved ones are suffering and traditional medicine doesn't seem to work. At the end of these conferences many people buy the speakers' books, visit their clinics and try their methods. Everybody remembers crobaiazin, a miracle cancer drug available mainly outside the United States: it took a long time and many scientific investigations to prove its ineffectiveness.

The point here is that if doctors want to serve their patients' best interests, they need to be both open-minded and vigilant against fraud.

TRADITION AND TREATMENT OF TERMINAL PATIENTS

Since my first year as a medical student I was always puzzled and worried whenever I approached a dying patient. How should I act? What should I say? For a naive and insecure medical student, dealing with dying patients was an enormous challenge. It's no less of a challenge to experienced physicians. While doctors' egos are inflated when they save patients' lives, their egos are deflated when they realized there's nothing they can do; they experience emotions ranging from humility to anger to denial.

From the beginning of my career, it struck me that there might be a better way of managing the care of dying patients. Physicians are so busy saving lives and curing diseases, they forget that a dying patient requires a different type of care. It's not unusual for a doctor to lose contact with a patient when he is dying. All too often, the patient is left on his own from the moment it becomes obvious he is dying.

It's not that doctors are heartless. Far from it. It's just that they're working within a healthcare system and a social culture that makes it difficult to respond to the real needs of dying patients. All the traditions and taboos create indifference at best and hostility, confusion and fear at worst. While friends, family and others all respond negatively and inappropriately to people who are dying, doctors have a greater opportunity to change their approach; they don't have the same emotional involvement with the patient as the family and could conceivably adopt a more humane method of treating these patients without all the other issues hampering their judgment. Unfortunately, doctors are bound by tradition and have difficulty challenging the status quo.

Forty years ago, the medical instructions for handling a dying patient were very simple. If the dying patient asked questions, the answer was that he was going through a difficult time at the moment but with the proper treatment he would soon be all right. If the patient brought up the question of death, the doctors and everyone else immediately reassured the patient that things were fine. As a result, the subject of impending death was never brought up. The doctor, on his daily rounds, acted confident around the dying patient and told him he was making progress. The nurses, family, and visitors similarly reassured the patient. The rationale behind this approach was that broaching the subject of death would unnecessarily upset the patient; he might not be able to handle it and even go so far as to commit suicide.

Here and in other countries, many doctors still follow this approach with minor variations. Because it's easily standardized and requires no effort or emotional strain from anyone surrounding the dying patient, this traditional strategy appeals to many healthcare professionals. It fails, however, to meet the highly individualized needs of dying patients as well as the evolving norms of medical care.

In terms of the later, the law has recently become strict and clear, resulting in the Patient's Bill of Rights. It states that before doctors treat ill patients, they must tell their patients in *easily understood language* (rather than obscure medical terminology):

The exact nature of their conditions.

The expected outcome.

The exact description of any medical or surgical procedure to be undertaken with the possible adverse outcome of each.

The alternative modes of treatment that can be considered.

Given these requirements, doctors cannot feign ignorance of a patient's true condition or pretend that things are better than they actually are.

Perhaps even more significantly, the traditional, standardized approach treats all patients as if they were the same. In reality, dying brings a patient's distinct personality into the light. Who a person is has a tremendous impact on how they deal with their dying. More than at any other time, doctors should be tailoring their approach to fit the patient. This is when patients need doctors to respond to who they are as individuals so that their individuality is acknowledged for the last time. Unfortunately, tradition does not grant doctors this degree of flexibility.

If there has been a break with tradition, it has come in the form of over-treatment of dying patients. Why would any doctor do too much for someone who is dying? Here are four reasons:

1. **The doctor's mission of maintaining life at all costs.** It has almost become an obsession. Doctors will routinely use extraordinary measures to keep a patient alive, especially if no one (such as the patient's family or the patient himself) tells the doctor to stop.

2. **Fear.** Fear comes in many forms, from a malpractice suit (because everything possible was not done for the patient, a suit might allege) to censure from colleagues or oversight committees.

3. **Ego.** This goes back to the doctor as a kind of god. As life-giver and life-saver, some doctors' egos get the better of their common sense. They overestimate their abilities as well as the technology at their disposal. As a result, they overtreat.

4. **Incentives.** Pharmaceutical and medical supply companies always have a new product they're pushing, and research departments always have a new drug or technique that is supposed to be a lifesaver and which is financed by generous grants. There are also more doctors than ever before who specialize in emergency medicine and perform emergency procedures on dying patients.

THE PROBLEMS WITH HOSPITAL POLICIES AND PROCEDURES

People cannot simply die of natural causes such as old age, general debilitation or organ failure in hospitals today. Instead, something or someone must be blamed. When a patient dies of a heart attack in an emergency room without being hooked up to a variety of machines, the death becomes suspicious ; it's sometimes difficult to prove that the death was not preventable. Death from widespread cancer metastasis and heart, kidney or pulmonary failure are thoroughly investigated. When these diseases are involved, there's always room for the argument that death could have been delayed even for a short time if a given procedure was performed. A death which occurs within thirty days after a patient leaves a hospital is examined to determine if mismanagement by the hospital was involved. All hospitals have a Mortality Review Committee that investigates every death that occurs within their walls.

There is nothing wrong with these committees in theory—it makes perfect sense to determine if a death was humanly preventable. The problem is that many of these committees fail to view the concept of preventable in context. Many deaths are preventable; life can be sustained for hours, days or even weeks with the right technology and treatment. But at what cost to the patient? Sometimes it's more humane to allow someone to die naturally than to prolong his agony.

I have witnessed discussions going on for hours in these committees where members argue about this notion of what's preventable. For instance, in the death of a ninety-year-old woman who came to the emergency room in a coma, the conclusion of the committee was that some procedure could have kept the comatose patient alive a little longer, and the death was classified preventable. Technically yes, but humanistically, no.

If you're uncertain about this last statement, walk through an emergency ward or Intensive Care Unit and see patients in comas or suffering from advanced terminal diseases hooked up to arterial or venous lines, with tubes placed through the throats, bladders, or various parts of their bodies to keep vital organs open. All this is extremely painful and of no benefit whatsoever since the terminally ill patient will die shortly anyway.

Review organizations responsible to the Department of Health, medical societies, and the hospitals themselves, are multiplying. To name a few, there are The Joint Commission of Hospitals, Utilization Review, Quality Insurance, Risk Management, Mortality Review, and Accident Prevention. Most of them help improve health care. At the same time, however, some of them turn dying into a bureaucratic nightmare that indirectly lowers the quality of life left to dying patients.

Many review organizations have overlapping functions, and some maintain their existence simply because they have created jobs, most of them well remunerated. To keep those jobs, people create strong, convincing justifications for them. Whether or not we need another layer of bureaucracy, we get it. It's very difficult for administrators who lack the necessary experience and expertise to make judgments about patients' deaths. Bureaucrats in the Department of Health, for instance, review all death certificates and rate any death that occurs in a hospital setting or at home within four weeks after discharge from a hospital, as a hospital death. These bureaucrats and their extensive staffs use some bizarre computer system, the mechanism of which is a mystery, to eliminate those that were, or almost were, dead on arrival, and then classify the hospitals by the percentage of deaths in relation to the number of admissions or the size of the hospital. All hospitals anxiously await the yearly publication of the report; it's like the triple-witching hour of the stock market. One year a hospital can be at the top of the list and the next year at the bottom. I have personally followed changes in the order of these ratings, and I can state with absolute certainty that it has nothing to do with magically improved medical care. It has to do with changing policies, procedures, and statistical manipulation.

If a dying patient is discharged a little early from the hospital because he wants to die at home surrounded by family, and if he stays alive for more than four weeks (terminal life can easily be extended at home through sedation and intravenous fluid administered by a visiting nurse), the hospital is deemed not to have killed the patient. My personal policy is that it is better to die at home surrounded by family than in a hospital setting. I, therefore, have removed many dying patients from the list of hospital deaths.

Hospitals usually have special and specific admission procedures whereby an admission to the emergency room (ER) is not necessarily a hospital admission, so that if a patient dies in the emergency room, it is not classified as a hospital death. Consequently, very sick patients are kept longer in the ER. Other hospitals put themselves on diversion either frequently or permanently, which means that patients cannot be admitted to their emergency rooms because of overload, and critical patients have to be diverted to other hospitals. Since the most qualified hospitals get the most seriously ill patients, they are punished by their high mortality rate, while the second-rate, smaller emergency rooms are rewarded for their low mortality rate by great-sounding mortality statistics.

Another policy to improve the mortality rate is to transfer sick patients. I know of a hospital that has a zero mortality rate for newborns. This would give the impression that all a pregnant woman has to do to make sure her baby is born alive and well is to give birth in that hospital. The truth is that any newborn with the slightest illness is immediately transferred to a more qualified institution, the statistics of which suffer accordingly.

Finally, ambulance drivers, who sometimes are bounced from one hospital to another because of overload capacity, have learned the hard way which hospitals to avoid and which ones are easily accessible. I know of a hospital with a back door entrance through which ambulance drivers can sneak in their emergency patients, thereby obliging the emergency room to treat the patient. Easily accessible hospitals with a modern and well-organized emergency room, qualified staff and up-to-date equipment are magnets for ambulance drivers who can quickly and safely unload their patients. They then leave to chase the next emergency patient since their job is to pick up and unload as many patients as possible during their shift. In these cases, ambulance drivers play an important role in increasing or decreasing the mortality rate of a hospital.

Lack of Expertise in Dealing With Terminal Patients

Just because a doctor has treated dying patients doesn't make him an expert on the subject. A doctor is only human and is subject to the same fear of death as anyone else. I have seen many doctors die, and I never saw one of them behave or react any differently than anyone outside the medical profession; they didn't have any inside knowledge about how to handle the situation. Denial of death is as common among physicians as it is among the general public. They are as afraid of death as anyone else. It's unfair for doctors to be perceived or present themselves as experts on dying. Years ago, family doctors could at least claim to know a patient well and have a sense of what the needs of that dying patient were. Today, the terminally ill patient is treated by a group of specialists and all too often the patient and family do not even know the physician in charge.

Invariably, however, people turn to the doctor for relief, understanding, and comfort when dealing with death. All too often, the terminally ill patient drags on for days and sometimes weeks in a coma or semi-coma, increasingly emaciated, barely able to move, and with the dreaded appearance of pre-death. All too often I have been approached privately by close family members and even by the patient when he was able to speak, asking me to stop the treatment and speed up or terminate the agony without any interference.

Doctors are increasingly perceived as experts in dying because they have become experts in extending life. We're living longer than ever before. Extended old age is a health hazard however, and, past middle age, there is hardly a human being not suffering from some defective organ, starting with backaches or other joint problems and terminating in progressive impairment of vital organs or systems of organs. We depend on doctors to keep us going as we live longer and experience one problem after another. Since they can successfully fix some of the problems we experience, why can't they fix all of them? Logically, we assume that a doctor who is an expert at extending life is also an expert at preventing and dealing with death.

There is a cultish aspect to this thinking, an almost religious mania to our fear of death. The priests of this new polytheism are various medical specialists. Not only does every patient of a particular age have a personal family doctor but also a list of personal specialists (cardiologist, gynecologist, urologist, gastroenterologist, ophthalmologist etc.), for various ailments. It is good practice to visit these new divinities frequently in their respective temples/offices, because like the Greco-Roman and Egyptian cultures there is a divinity for each and every specific medical condition.

Doctors used to be relatively humble creatures. Today, many physicians act as if they are divine and all-powerful. Because we have become an increasingly atheistic or agnostic culture, we reflexively look for someone to worship, and doctors are the logical candidates for that role. Whether they've had the role thrust upon them or created this divine image themselves, is beside the point. What's important is that no human being can live up to it. When a doctor doesn't perform the expected miracle, people lose faith in the doctor but they don't lose faith in the concept of doctor as miracle-worker. They simply look for another specialist to worship.

Some doctors have tried to return to a more appropriate, mortal role, but they're often rebuffed in these efforts. For instance, when a physician refuses to treat—or rather when he has no lifesaving measure to offer a dying patient—he may be accused of withdrawing from the case or even of withholding treatment. To help the patient approach death with dignity and without pain or anxiety is becoming difficult (ACOG Committee Opinion, Committee on Ethics, Number 158, May 1995).

How can doctors and hospitals help patients achieve a more human death? As we'll see, a radical and even revolutionary approach is required.

Chapter 9

THE FUNERAL INDUSTRY:
RESPONDING TO THE EMOTIONAL NEEDS OF THE LIVING

Memento quia pulvis es. Remember that you are only dust and that you will return to earth. −Quotation from the Bible

Jessica Milford and others have written about the American way of death and the abuses of the funeral industry. My goal here isn't to repeat those charges but to give you another perspective on why the funeral industry contributes to the negative aspects of dying in our culture. As you'll see, they are no more culpable than the families and friends of the dying who encourage them to make the process more irritating and unnatural than it needs to be.

THE TRADITIONAL ROLES OF RELIGIOUS FIGURES

In previous generations, the care of both the dying and the dead was almost exclusively handled by religious authorities. In this capacity, they had the following two roles:

1. Assisting terminally ill patients to pass from this world to the next. Responsibilities attached to this role included confession, Extreme Unction for Catholics, theological discussions on the uncertainties of this life and the certainty of afterlife and writing a will. Clergy were also responsible for orchestrating a final farewell, a ceremonial leave-taking that allowed the dying person to be involved in a larger event rather than terribly alone.

2. Taking care of the dead body and the bereaved family. From the moment of death to the end of the mourning period, religious authorities supervised the formal burial and mourning process. They didn't distinguish between taking care of the dying and the dead.

Increasingly, the clergy abandoned these two roles. In terms of the former, I've discussed how the medical professional has largely taken over managing the transition from this world to the next. The funeral industry has taken over the second role. Many years ago, morticians limited themselves to carpentry, making large, simple boxes of wood to carry the body from home to the church and then to the cemetery for burial. Gradually, however morticians became funeral directors and assumed much more responsibility for an increasingly complex series of tasks. They now assume an almost quasi-religious aura as they coordinate and control what happens until the body is buried in the ground.

MEETING A DEEPER NEED

It is difficult to understand the underlying power of the funeral industry unless one is aware that they fill important social and emotional needs. To understand how they do so, consider how the comforting words spoken by clergy to the dying and at funerals have changed. Today there is often not much said about an afterlife; it is almost embarrassing to mention it. The emphasis now is on the memory of the person who has died. Funeral orations by the clergy usually address accomplishments during life, bereavement of the family and how the departed shall be remembered by the living.

The memory left behind is what counts, and this is where the funeral industry steps in. Funeral directors help satisfy their clients' goal of a lasting memory. This is rather easy since, contrary to the clergy and/or medical profession, they are not (and are careful not to be) connected with the painful process of dying. It is easy to offer comfort when you do not have to explain a doubtful afterlife as the clergy does or to account for death as physicians do. They simply offer a lasting memory of the deceased, a ceremony as elaborate as money can buy. They pick up the pieces of a tragedy that is already underway and offer comfort. They craft a beautiful image of the deceased through a beautiful ceremony, functioning in the following seven ways:

Function #1: Taking Charge. After the doctor has pronounced someone dead, the family is stricken with anguish and does not know what to do. Confused and distracted, they are confronted by a series of decisions about the death certificate, what to do with the body, how to make arrangements for the funeral or the burial, how to list and notify friends and relatives and so on. One phone call to the funeral chapel, however, and these decisions are lifted like a great burden from their shoulders. The funeral chapel will immediately send a dignified and compassionate agent (grief therapist) to the home to familiarize the responsible member of the family with all the procedures: "Just sign here, please.

Function #2: Removal of the body. Funeral homes are eager to do this quickly because once they accomplish this task, it means they are officially in charge. The funeral director, an excellent grief therapist, also knows that the presence of the body at home or even in the hospital is unbearable for the family. Gone are the days when family members took turns sitting close with the body overnight until it was removed to the church for the funeral ceremony or directly to the cemetery. It has almost been forgotten that the original purpose of this custom was to make sure the deceased was effectively dead since there was no scientific way to pronounce death and one had to wait until the mask of death (immobile and pale face with characteristic features) appeared.

Function #3: Embalming. Funeral directors capitalized on our dread of death and fear of this mask by introducing embalming—a procedure that removes this mask. Embalming is the reason they give for removing the body as quickly as possible. The funeral director knows only too well that a body with a peaceful face reposing in a beautiful casket makes death more acceptable and certainly is more appealing than a face that shows the struggle that preceded death.

Contrary to myth, embalming has no sanitary purpose and does not prevent a body from decaying. Very few people know that embalming is not required by law. Its real purpose is to beautify the face of the deceased through subcutaneous injection of different materials in the facial blood vessels; carefully applied makeup adds to the effect.

When the face bears a beatific look, the deceased seems to be at peace and resting in eternity. Again, this relates to the larger goal of leaving mourners with a lasting memory.

Function #4: The Casket. The way the casket appears has become as important as the appearance of the body itself. Funeral directors offer a first class seat for the final voyage. This is their money-back guarantee of a beautiful and lasting memory. "Ashes to ashes, dust to dust, earth to earth" is over. The custom of placing the body in a shroud for burial in a grave where it eventually returns to the earth has been completely abandoned. The idea of worms eating the dead body is dreadful, and the funeral industry erased it thoroughly. Now the casket, containing a mattress covered with silk and satin and a beautiful pillow on which the deceased's head can comfortably rest, is the norm. An elaborate, hermetically sealed, casket offers the illusion that a body will be preserved for eternity. In reality, it is doubtful that the body lasts any longer in a casket than if it were buried directly in the earth. The sanitary function of a casket is also unfounded because burying a body in a grave poses no threat of spreading any disease.

Function #5: Flowers. Flowers and elaborate floral arrangements have become a must for any funeral. The floral industry works hand in hand with the funeral industry because they both have a similar goal: Making the funeral ceremony as elaborate as possible to make the memory as beautiful and lasting as possible.

Function #6: Religious ceremony. Funeral directors never antagonize the clergy and will make all the arrangements necessary for conducting the religious aspect of the funeral. They will even propose a religious minister to the family if they do not have one. They recognize that though the religious aspect of mourning is now largely de-emphasized, a religious service lends a formality and structure that helps them craft a memory.

Function #7: A funeral parlor as beautiful as a wedding chapel.
It used to be that the funeral ceremonies took place in the deceased's family's home or graveside. The former, however, often is too small and ordinary for this type of event and the latter is too depressing and subject to inclement weather. The church too, has fallen out of favor with many because issues such as an afterlife and heaven and hell seem too old-fashioned. Funeral chapels and parlors, on the other hand, have become very successful primarily because they liberated the family from any regulations or restrictions imposed by the church or cemetery. In other words, they allow people the freedom to tailor the ceremony to their particular needs. The funeral industry organizes the ceremony to please their clients unlike the church or the cemetery.

Many additional advantages are found in funeral parlors. They always offer a room where visitors gather to express their sympathy to the grieving family. These gatherings can last for several hours, allowing social contacts to be established and renewed. Snobbery can be displayed by the exhibition of an expensive casket, flowers, and other aspects of the ceremony. This display of wealth also can express the guilt frequently felt by the family: "The least we can do for him now is provide the most beautiful funeral money can buy." The funeral director plays on this guilt. The funeral ceremony at the funeral chapel or parlor has become so customary that it is almost mandatory and a family would be considered odd not to conform.

We Get What We Ask (and Pay) For

It is easy to scapegoat the funeral industry for the problems associated with the high cost of dying and the obscene elaborateness of the funeral ceremony. Conservative clergy have certainly attacked the lavish display in funeral parlor ceremonies and would like a return to a more humble treatment of death rather than what they refer to as the paganistic rituals. The funeral industry also comes to loggerheads with the medical profession on occasion because autopsies and tissue removal for transplants interfere with embalming. Cremation is becoming popular and is making embalming unnecessary. In additional, turf wars sometimes flare up between the funeral industry and cemeteries over who is responsible for what functions. On top of all this, the press is screaming louder and louder about the escalating cost of dying.

While some funeral directors commit abuses and capitalize on the confusion, grief, guilt, and snobbery of the family to extract the maximum profit, they are not the villains in this morality play. Like any other business, they exist to make money, and most funeral parlors compete within legal boundaries. The notion of governmental or other controls on the industry seems like a gross overreaction.

It is instructive, however, to discuss the underlying issues raised by the funeral industry's goal of providing lasting memories. Clemenceau, the French Prime Minister who led his country to victory during World War I, was famous for saying: "People have the kind of government they deserve." Paraphrasing this statement, I would add that we have the type of funerals we ask for. Some critics are appalled by the huge amount of money wasted on flowers—billions of dollars annually, if the estimates can be believed. My question is, why not? I have never heard of flower shops soliciting families to spend money on flowers for funerals the way they solicit them to spend money on flowers for weddings, anniversaries, or other occasions. When a close friend passes away, I invariably go to the flower shop to select an arrangement, and I have never seen the name of a flower shop advertised in a funeral parlor.

Similarly, some people choose to spend a great deal of money on caskets, funeral ceremonies and the like. Whether they do so out of love, guilt or snobbishness, this is their issue, and it seems unfair to blame the funeral industry for responding to their requests. It would be just as unfair to attack a luxury automobile company because people choose to drive an expensive car or a real estate company that sells a large house. We live in an affluent society, and affluence is expressed in different ways. In some families, wealth is displayed with no thought to the wishes of the deceased, just as in some weddings, the parents display their wealth without consideration of the bride and groom's wishes.

There's a lesson to be learned from the way in which we turn funerals into photo opportunities; for the manner in which we create lasting memories. Funeral directors are brilliant grief therapists; they know how desperate mourners are for these memories and how their fear of death drives this desperation. They know that the fear of death is at its highest point during the funeral and that many mourners are almost in a trance, concerned with a sudden and irrevocable plunge into an abyss, completely disoriented, and with limited or no hope of creating a lasting memory. Funeral directors also know that the doctors and clergy are not going to relieve the family's anxieties.

The greatest achievement of the funeral directors is to transform, through embalming, a dead body on the way to decay into a serene body at eternal peace to the great relief of the family. I will never forget the case of a colleague's spouse, who proudly exhibited the face of her dead husband (after embalming) in the funeral parlor. In retrospect it may seem grotesque, but to her it was a tremendous relief. She had her memory, and to a certain extent her fear was reduced (because her husband did not look much different in death from the way he looked in life—it was easy to believe that he had been preserved and would not physically fade away).

Funeral directors are professionals, and as such they relieve anxiety because they seem to understand what to do about death better than the rest of us. The personnel in the funeral parlor are sure of themselves; they have appropriate answers for all the problems associated with death. They act as counselors and advisers.

The way in which we turn to funeral directors for advice points out the tremendous vacuum in our society when it comes to dealing with dying and death. Even the most well-meaning and knowledgeable funeral director can only provide superficial assistance. Still, funeral directors are whom most people turn for help. Certainly the clergy and doctors aren't filling this role in a meaningful way.

Rather than criticize the funeral industry for its excesses, we should focus on our own fears and needs. It makes perfect sense that each of us should dictate how we want our funeral to be handled ahead of time. The problem, of course, is that people do leave instructions in this regard that are often ignored by the family. Perhaps we need legislation to enforce the funeral wishes of the dying. Until that time, family, friends, customs, traditions, funeral industry policies and other factors will contribute to the expensive and elaborate funerals that are commonplace today. Unless we get past our fear of death and our need for one last perfect memory, funerals will continue to be conducted to meet the emotional needs of survivors rather than the deceased.

A Ludicrous Process in Need of Change

Funerals temporarily relieve the fear felt by those close to the person who died. The funeral industry expertly orchestrates the process so that the initial terror that threatens to overwhelm people after someone dies quickly is transformed into happiness and laughter. If you've ever gone to a funeral parlor to view the remains, you are aware of how somber the mood is and how many tears are shed. Then people hug the surviving family and whisper words of solace and bereavement. Few people look at the deceased, terrified that they are looking at their own fate at some point in the future. After this, however, the funeral ceremony makes the transition from somber to social. Conversations are struck, new people are introduced and soon the talk is about everything except death. In fact, if you didn't know someone had just died, you would think you were at a wonderful party. Everyone is laughing, drinking and eating. Then people get in their cars and become part of an elaborate funeral procession to the cemetery; with headlamps on and the freedom to drive through red lights, the procession resembles a parade.

The whole process puts a band-aid on grieving. Instead of allowing people to air their feelings and grievances, the party and parade are distractions. No one is allowed to talk about their own fear of death. The funeral industry has institutionalized this process and profited from it. They have no interest in changing it.

Fortunately, some people are forcing them to change. Adverse publicity certainly is a factor in these changes. In addition, friends of the deceased or clergy take an intermediary role and arrange for the funeral. These intermediaries often are sufficiently knowledgeable about the process that they can reduce or eliminate some of the excessive practices and charges. They can also help tailor the funeral so that it meets the expressed desires of the person who died.

Still, the funeral directors aren't the only ones who deserve blame. They are simply responding to the market as any good business person would. It's up to us to start addressing our own fears and understand how they're the real cause of all absurdities of the funeral process.

Chapter 10

THE TRANSITION FROM RELIGION-MANAGED
TO MEDICAL-MANAGED DEATH

Historical analysis gives us insights into how and why we believe what we do about death. Without this historical perspective, we jump to conclusions—often false conclusions. It helps to understand that our current approach to dying and death evolved out of a series of events and beliefs, and that what evolved is not necessarily the right approach.

Knowledge provides us with a broader frame of reference in which to think about a situation. When we remove the mystery from our current practices regarding the dead, we can look at these practices more objectively. We can also become more open-minded about alternatives to the status quo.

Let's begin our historical analysis by considering the five different ways people view life after death and how these perspectives evolved. In this chapter we will concentrate on Western history; the next chapter will describe specific aspects of Eastern culture.

Six Types of Afterlife

People think about the afterlife in strikingly different ways. Here are the six most common perceptions:

1. **No life or existence after death.** Atheism endorses this notion, and it has gained many adherents over the years. Agnostics or even those who have some religious affiliation may lean toward this view.

2. **Memory after death**. As we've discussed earlier, the notion of a persistent memory is one in which we remain in the minds of those who have known us, especially our family, friends and colleagues. Some leave a lasting memory represented by earthly accomplishments while a few achieve a larger measure of fame.

3. **Existence of life beyond earth in terrestrial terms.** We are physically transported to a religious paradise or hell. This viewpoint is losing favor in most religions and countries; the idea of a cosmic existence is usually integrated with this paradisial place.

4. **Cosmic existence.** A pure and abstract existence, detached from one's body as well as from space, time, familiar surroundings and even consciousness. While on earth, we can prepare for this new kind of existence, especially in old age, by learning to separate from our attachments and learn to perceive the beyond.

5. **Reincarnation.** Our soul was in someone else before our birth and will go to someone else after we die. This concept is more common than one might imagine and is not necessarily religious in nature. Some cultures believe they are reincarnated in their children while others believe they come back as animals.

6. **Blocking the subject.** Some people become very nervous when the subject is discussed and prefer not to talk about it.

The Historical Shaping of Our Perceptions

Until the Middle Ages ended and the Renaissance began (end of the 15th century), civilized people had an almost uniform belief in life after death. God, heaven and hell and the idea of death as a passage from one condition to the next were widely accepted except for a few intellectual skeptics. While the concept of an afterlife varied among different religious groups, it was always present and automatically accepted.

Before Christianity, the belief was that the body and soul together were transferred to an afterlife. There was, therefore, respect for the dead body which was considered the carrier even after death. Ceremonies revolved around this belief, perhaps the most well-known ones being the embalming of the corpse and the construction of the pyramids for the Pharaohs of ancient Egypt. With the advent of Christianity, people began viewing the body and soul as separate entities. The biological demands of the body (food, sex, etc.) were considered handicaps for the movement of the soul. Although people enjoyed themselves during their lifetimes, this enjoyment was considered almost sinful. Death was nothing more than the liberation of the soul from the body and the soul went to heaven (or hell or purgatory). The Christian dying ceremony represented the detachment of the soul from the body and all of its sinful pleasures. The dead body was no longer viewed as a carrier and became less important. It was nothing more than a reminder, a symbol, of the departed person.

Until the end of the Middle Ages, each event in the universe was considered a divine miracle. Everything was a miraculous event: day and night, sunrise and sunset, the seasons, plants, animals, life, and birth. Given this perspective, even death possessed a miraculous aura. To question whether death might simply be a sleep from which one did not awake was almost inconceivable. Without a scientific explanation, death and other events were elevated far beyond the status to which scientific thought reduced them. Given the miracles all around people, being religious was as natural as breathing. Religious leaders didn't spend their time attempting to convince people of the existence of God; everyone knew it to be true. Instead, the priests were involved in teaching a specific form of belief and a specific way of life according to the will of a specific God. The adversaries of a religion were not atheists or nonbelievers but those who deviated from the specific teaching of a given religion and altered its well-delineated dogma. To convert someone to a religion was not to convert a nonbeliever to a believer but to transfer someone from the dogma of one religion to the dogma of another. It should be noted that the term, evangelize , originally meant to substitute Christianity for Paganism; it connoted a change of religions.

Throughout ancient history, there were a few isolated rebellions against these beliefs such as the rational thinking of the Greek philosophers. But the all-powerful church quickly put down these rebellions. Tools such as the Inquisition also discouraged any deviation from the norm. Even medicine was under the authority of the church and some medical schools of the Middle Ages were run by the clergy. Doctors were not responsible for death and people died because God called them to join Him. Unless it was an obvious criminal act (stabbing, poisoning, etc.) death, specifically a slow, disease-induced death, was always an act of God.

It was only at the end of the Middle Ages that doubt about an afterlife started to creep in. This transformation in thought, which started at the beginning of the 16th century, was widespread by the 19th century, at least in the Western World. Though there are still people who believe in an afterlife, doubt always exists. Religious leaders today, unlike those before the 16th century, labor mightily to convince people of divine existence. This change says a lot about how our beliefs have been transformed.

We've also become very skeptical of miracles, and religious belief has a rather narrow connotation, meaning that one believes in some kind of modus operandi in the universe that has no physical or scientific explanation. A religious person believes in events that are in opposition to the laws of a biological and physical world. It's rare today to find some event that is not scientifically explained and which would imply a divine (or demonic) presence.

The change from belief to non-belief probably took a couple of centuries, and it was catalyzed by scientific explanations for an increasing number of previously unexplained phenomenon. Everything in the universe, such as sunrise and sunset and rain or drought, received a scientific explanation instead of being accepted as divine miracles. The body started to be better understood in terms of its physiology and pathology. Death was understood in terms of physiological failures that could sometimes be corrected. As skepticism about afterlife continued to creep in, death became a horror and discussing it became frightening because it signified the end of everything. Not only was it frightening to elderly people but to anyone as they aged. Even the clergy started to talk less about death and only spoke of absolution and heaven (much less of hell). They didn't have answers to those dreaded questions about death; it was better to keep those questions buried in the subconscious than allow them to surface. I imagine the clergy themselves were too frightened and confused by their own doubts and were eager to drop the subject of death (Ariès, 1982).

THE DOCTOR'S DILEMMA:

As doctors gradually freed themselves from the powerful grip of the Church, they had more opportunities to use real science to investigate causes of disease and determine treatment. Instead of relying on prayers, they could put their science to work. At first, this was a radical departure from tradition, since doctors were burned at the stake in the Middle Ages for separating medicine from religion.

But the opportunities afforded by this new medical freedom also came with a price: It was no longer God's will if the treatment failed; rather, it was the doctor's failure. Now the doctor, not God, became the maker of life and death. Over time, doctors became the managers of death and dying, a role the clergy was more than eager to turn over to them. When someone was dying, a doctor was called before or even instead of the priest. Unfortunately, doctors didn't have as much experience dealing with dying people that the clergy had developed over the centuries. The clergy had been carefully taught, during their priesthood training, how to interact with the dying and their skilled manner was always a comfort. Doctors lacked this training. Even more troublesome, doctors weren't allowed to talk about afterlife since it was unscientific, unproved and irrational. For doctors as well as patients, death had become a dreaded subject, one that was difficult to discuss at all.

To talk or not to talk about death, that was the question and the dilemma facing doctors. For most the 17th, 18th and 19th centuries, doctors didn't resolve this dilemma. Instead, they avoided the subject as much as possible. Without the training or experience, they managed the deaths of their patients uncertainly and inconsistently.

By the beginning of the 20th century, however, doctors took a new approach: They decided to rebel against death and fight it until the bitter end. This rebellion would have been considered sacrilegious during the Middle Ages. Today, however, it has become medical dogma. While extending life is a noble goal, it ceases to be noble when the life that is extended is filled with suffering. Extending life at any cost has more in common with the tortures of the Inquisition than the wise and compassionate use of modern science.

Through gerontology, doctors have learned to extend life into very old age, resulting in a significant percentage of senior citizens who are completely bedridden and mentally deficient. This country now has 50,000 centenarians, a few healthy but most suffering from varying degrees of physical or mental defects. Using science to sustain the lives of terminally ill and elderly people is a worthy goal if the following criteria are kept in mind:

1. Patients should not be used as guinea pigs to test new or experimental treatments.

2. The life-extending treatments should not be motivated by our fear of death.

3. Treatment should be in response to the patient's desire to be kept alive rather than someone else's wish (or fear).

Unfortunately, these criteria are often ignored as the entire healthcare industry—doctors, nurses, administrators, hospitals, HMOs—has joined the fight against death. Advances in medical care, medical technology, pharmacology, and medical equipment have been aimed at extended life. In this zealous quest to add hours or days to a person's life, what gets lost are quality of life issues. Historical progress in medicine may be easier to measure in quantitative terms—in the amount of time we can extend lives through modern medicine—but the true measure is improving the quality of life.

How the Medical Profession Took Over the Mortuary Function

As mentioned in previous chapters, the price of consciousness and of superior thinking that characterizes humans is the awareness that one is alive as well as that one is dying. Since the dawn of mankind, humans have struggled unsuccessfully with how to die and what happens to us after death. The relief and comfort offered by religion was temporary and is now vanishing. Almost by default, the medical profession has taken over this role of reliever and comforter. In reality, doctors have no training whatsoever to deal with these issues. They are taught how to save lives and not how to help people when they're dying.

If doctors are going to perform this role effectively—and I am not sure they should—then they need special training and a completely different attitude.

How the medical profession got involved in the pre-mortuary and mortuary function is a mystery of the evolution of medicine into which historians of the next generation will try to delve. The most mystifying aspect is that today it has become so natural that no one finds anything mysterious about it.

Presently, when the question of possible death arises, when someone is dying, when someone presents any problem while dying, when someone is pronounced dead, when the news is to be announced to the family, when it comes to the family's bereavement, and even the administrative papers associated with death (death certificate), the medical profession is asked to handle everything. Not only is it a mystery to me that everyone finds this medical function natural, but that the doctor also finds it natural, and most often the doctor "does something." From a medical point of view this means nothing, since the patient dies anyway. Under these conditions, to do something often ends up being harmful.

Chapter 11

RELIGIOUS DIFFERENCES:
WHERE EAST DOESN'T MEET WEST

"I will believe in the existence of the soul, when I see it at the tip of my scalpel" –Popular Quotation among Atheist Scientists

As human intelligence started to emerge, primitive man needed some explanation to account for the universe around him. The most logical and simple explanation was to see the universe under the control of supernatural power(s). From the beginning, it was thought that various supernatural powers were controlling what took place on earth. A different divinity existed for everything that had to be explained. Later, with Judaism, Christianity, and Islam, the concept of monotheism became dominant.

The terrible fear and anxiety produced by death would largely disappear if we all had irrefutable proof of an afterlife. In lieu of that proof, we have religion, and for many years, it sufficed. It's only in modern times that religion has offered less comfort in this regard. As a result, people in Western cultures fight death until the last dying gasp and exacerbate rather than alleviate fear of that final moment. Before attempting to define a new approach to death, let us discuss how different the approach to death is in other cultures.

Interestingly, people in Eastern cultures traditionally experience less anxiety and fear than do people in the West. Their religions and attitudes about death have somehow fostered greater acceptance of death and dying. Consequently, people in Eastern countries are prone to die more peacefully—and with far less guilt, anger and other negative emotions—than people in Western cultures.

It's instructive to examine the contrast in cultures and how this contrast evolved over time. By looking at the different approaches to death, we can see that there's at least one viable alternative to our own.

Nothing fueled the growth of religion more than the way in which religious beliefs relieved innate human anxieties about death. The notion of life after death was enormously appealing, and it's what made early Christianity so attractive to the slaves of the Roman Empire. Certainly the promise of an afterlife was far more appealing than their earthly life. All that was required was belief, and the reward for that belief was heaven.

The notion of the soul going to Heaven was used by political and religious authorities to move people in specific directions. From the Crusades to the Iran-Iraq conflict, wars have been religiously motivated or related in some way to religious belief. Religious leaders frequently contrasted the uncertainties of life (disease, accidents, etc.) with the idea of heaven. Thinking about and aspiring to this blissful afterlife became a constant in people's lives. One could take refuge in it and find it more appealing than an often brutal existence. Christianity always stressed the dead and the dying as candidates for Heaven. Resignation and even courage marked the passage from this life to the next, and there was rarely a rebellion against it. Instead, calm acceptance was the rule. There was the sense that one did not die but went to rest, and that this rest was badly needed.

By the time of the Crusades, however, doubt probably began to alter this religious perspective. The Crusaders were shocked to see that God was not with them in liberating the Holy Land and, in fact, they were beaten by these unbelievers who appeared to be very comfortable with a different faith. These Crusaders brought back a new, more skeptical way of thinking. Could there be another God besides the Crusaders' God? Or, maybe there was no God. This skepticism called the idea of life after death into question.

Astronomers, such as Copernicus, taking a chance on being burned alive as heretics, presented a universal system somehow at variance with the teaching of the Bible. Physicians such as Ambroise Paré and mathematicians and physicists such as Leonardo da Vinci and many others made tremendous progress in describing the universe. Descartes (1596) in Discourse on Method introduced the concept of doubt about any proposition and was essentially the founder of basic scientific observation. The theory of evolution (Darwin, 1859; Wallace, 1858) dealt a final blow to orthodox thinking. No aspect of the universe, no matter how big or small, was immune from scientific analysis. Science has presented, or at least proposed, an explanation for practically every mystery of the universe, in terms of astronomy, cosmology, biology, zoology, oceanography, geography, geology, archeology, anthropology, medicine, etc. Many questions remain unanswered, but sound theories for understanding the whole universe in space and time were posited and communicated to the masses. The combination of computers and genetics has given the world the sense that we (rather than a higher power) control our destiny.

Progress in medicine was made thanks to careful anatomical observations and important physiological and biological discoveries. From very early on, physicians felt confident in proposing cures for almost everything. In the beginning, physicians received tremendous help from the placebo effect. The body carries within itself the possibility of self cure and spontaneous healing, and so a wound or a fracture frequently heals spontaneously. Any treatment (or lack thereof) proposed during the spontaneous cure was given credit for the cure. It was only with the introduction of surgery, anesthesia, antisepsis, transfusions, fluid and electrolyte balance, antibiotics, radiology, medical subspecialties and other treatments that medicine really became curative, and even then the placebo effect still played a significant role.

At first, organized religion was hostile toward science. In the beginning, the church considered science to be witchcraft, a tool of the devil. Over time, however, church leaders recognized that scientific discoveries and religious tenets could be compatible. Today, religion takes a more philosophical attitude (Teilhard de Chardin, 1964), and the traditional hostility toward science and scientific discoveries has largely dissipated.

Given all the scientific progress that has been made and mysteries revealed, it is important to note that only one mystery remains where science is at a loss for an explanation. Science has been unable to provide any proof of life after death. Certainly this is a difficult concept for anyone to get their mind around. Where is the other world to which our mind, body and spirit goes? The cosmos has been explored enough to convince everyone that heaven has not been located. It may be incredibly hot miles beneath the earth's surface, but science suggests that all that's down there is heat, not hell. Scientific evidence opposes the concept of a world where a dead person will go, at least in the ordinary concept of a world existing in space and time where one would exist physically or mentally after death.

Today, philosophy and even modern religions speak of life after death in a more abstract form. The abstract notion of an afterlife may satisfy a few intellectuals, but it's not much solace for most people who believe that nothing exists after death or that the possibility of life after death is a longshot. Thus, our fear. Nothing has replaced the comfort religion used to provide.

Unfortunately, we have been unable to create a philosophy or practices that are an adequate substitute for religion as death approaches. While some people still desperately turn to religion as they're dying, they do so out of panic; they're grasping at straws. While science may enable people to live longer, it does not help them die better.

A Spiritual Vacuum in Western Culture

In all the modern medical books I have read concerning the management of dying patients, religion is never mentioned; the possibility of heaven and hell are ignored. It strikes me that even psychoanalysis and psychotherapy largely ignore it. The reasoning behind this omission must be that because there is no scientific proof of God, the devil and heaven and hell, these subjects are irrelevant to any scientific study.

At the same time, however, these religious issues are very much on the minds of those who are dying. Most people have been exposed to some religion as children. Even if they didn't practice their religion as adults, their early religious experiences often take on new power as their lives draw to a close. It is second nature for people to look toward religion as they lay dying; it has been this way for thousands of years.

Families aren't always aware of this impulse. On a number of occasions, I've seen dying patients who lived largely non-religious lives shock their families by requesting a visit from a minister, priest or rabbi. Neither family nor healthcare professionals should underestimate the power of this impulse. I've seen many dying people gain real peace from religious absolution and forgiveness. There are no atheists in foxholes. In a cynical, atheistic age, highly religious people may seem hopelessly naive and overly hard on themselves. But they gain a measure of revenge (if revenge is the appropriate term) when they die secure in the knowledge that they have lived good lives and will go to heaven.

In earlier centuries, the coming of death always entailed a discussion of the world beyond. Religion catalyzed this discussion, and the focus was much more on what came after death than the dying process. Today, however, the situation is reversed. In the absence of a strong religious conviction, talk of death revolves around the possibility of nothingness and the horror of non-existence. It's no wonder that people flee from this sort of conversation with someone who is dying. But without any discussion of this topic, the dying individual feels terribly isolated and alone.

As different as world religions are from one another, just about all of them share a belief in a life after death. Though Judaism did not originally mention an afterlife (the Old Testament does not mention it at all), the prophets were emphatic about it. Islam is very insistent that the life beyond this one is far superior. For American Indians, to die with courage and to be strong in suffering was the surest way to go to paradise.

As religious belief has lost its power over people, we find ourselves in a dangerous vacuum of purely rational thought. Rationalization does not diminish the fear of death; we cannot find anything good or useful to justify losing our lives. Which is why we're incredulous when we hear about people in Asia or other Eastern cultures who accept death without the massive resistance that is embedded in western societies.

141

The Alternative Offered by Eastern Culture

In many Eastern countries, death is considered a culmination, an accomplishment, a condition one steps into after struggling with the obstacles of this world and a well-deserved reward after a full life. Easterners reach a point when they no longer wish to participate in the activities of life; they no longer wish to see, hear, touch, eat, drink, or wake up and continue their daily existence. Modern philosophers might refer to this phenomenon as an unwillingness to participate in the concept of space and time. I simply call it no longer wishing to be <u>conscious</u> of life. After death, Easterners see themselves born into a new world that challenges, defies, and is different from our present world of space, time and consciousness.

This Eastern mindset has three distinct advantages as death approaches:

1. Rather than being obsessed about not leaving this life, they are looking forward to leaving it.

2. They don't agonize over the type of existence they'll have after death.

3. They reject a conscious and individual existence after death and conceive of it only in unconscious or non-conscious terms.

This last point probably is the one that's most important in helping them leave this life peacefully. From the Eastern perspective, the afterlife is a state in which one becomes fused with other dead people and no longer exist individually. In this state, consciousness is not only unnecessary but a burden. It's important to emphasize that this perception isn't built from logic, experience and deduction. Instead, it is felt more than explained, sensed more than perceived and derationalized more than rationalized. It is a very democratic philosophy, at least in the sense that it is accessible to all people and not only the most educated (Evans-Wentz, 1960). In the Eastern world, preparation for death is a prolonged meditative process that starts early in life or at least well before one's final days. As Easterners advance in age they talk more freely about approaching death.

As you can see, this Eastern approach is in direct conflict with our Western view. Part of the conflict has to do with our affluent society. In a world of material wealth, death is especially painful because you can't take it with you. The loss of things accumulated over time is painful. We have lived such a comfortable existence, it's difficult to leave it. We find the mere mention of death off-putting and we don't even like to think about it. As a result, we don't prepare ourselves for the inevitable end of life. When death nears, it is always a catastrophe, a drama that unexpectedly takes everyone (the dying and surrounding people) by surprise and is dealt with awkwardly and even ignorantly. Mismanaging death goes hand-in-hand with this awkwardness and ignorance. Even if the dying process is slow (as with terminal cancer) and there is time to prepare, death is always sudden in the sense that the time is used to fight death rather than prepare for it.

In Eastern culture, elderly people may spend years in an extended ceremony preparing for their deaths. As soon as people become sick and people recognize that sooner or later they will die from their illness, they begin a ritual of preparation. In fact, in some Asian countries, funeral homes often function as the best place to hospitalize and care for a terminally ill patient who has reached a comatose or pre-comatose state. Nothing is done for these terminal patients except to wait for them to die, and the family (or some member) waits in the parlor until someone comes to announce the person is dead. To interfere with death is almost sacrilegious. From an Eastern perspective, the frenetic activity of our emergency rooms and the heroic procedures used to sustain life for days or weeks is heresy. It is interference with a natural and inexorable process.

I recall watching a family of recent Asian immigrants bring an elderly member about to die to our modern emergency room. They assumed the dying person had been brought to a pre-funeral parlor where the staff would simply observe and allow him to die peacefully. Instead, they were shocked to see our hysterical and frantic efforts as we resuscitated the patient and kept him alive with all kinds of medications and intervention equipment. Then the patient, barely hanging on to life, was discharged in the family's care, and the family was given instructions on how to use medications, procedures and equipment to keep the patient alive. Within a week, the family returned to the emergency room as the patient, suffering terribly, almost died again. The emergency room team worked another miracle and managed to prolong the patient's life for another two days. This Asian family eventually receives a huge bill for all this medical care and eventually the threat of legal action unless the bill is paid promptly.

It's a rude awakening for people from the East who view the dying process as ceremonial and a peaceful voyage from one world to the next. But it's also a seductive vision—the notion that death can be fought off—and Western influence has caused many Eastern people to discard their old beliefs in favor of our more modern ones.

Death with dignity is a phrase that is slowly gaining favor in the West as we realize that modern is not necessarily better. Though we still have a long way to go before we make death with dignity a widespread reality, we should take a cue from Eastern culture where death with dignity is a way of life. The family respects the condition of each dying individual, and no one forces them to cling to life. Certainly Eastern people feel grief for those who die because they miss them, but they don't feel pity for them; they realize that the dead have gone on to a different if not a better world. Interference with death is minimal, only if the dying person wishes it, and only if it reestablishes life with dignity. It is not a temporary and distorted way of life without dignity or an insult to the deceased and family.

Hindus recoil at Western concepts of extending life in ways that compromise the quality of life. To them, human interference with death is a sacrilege, artificially postponing the nature cycle of afterlife and reincarnation. They view suicide as the same sort of heresy since it constitutes interference in the natural order of things. At the same time, Hindus support pain control and euthanasia because they encourage focused religious thought at the moment of death. Spiritual enlightenment is at the core of the Hindu belief system, and pain control and euthanasia make it possible for people to experience this enlightenment as they are dying.

Buddhists and Taoists also place a strong emphasis on spiritual peace at the time of death, believing that it will facilitate rebirth. It's not unusual for family members to chant at the bedside of someone who is dying. They also accept the use of medication when someone is in extreme pain. It's interesting to note that these Eastern religions, unlike primitive Christianity, have always believed that suffering interferes with rather than promotes spiritual liberation. They are not burdened with the image of Christ dying on the cross and the concomitant belief that there is a noble aspect to suffering.

Another common belief in Eastern religions is reincarnation when, at the time of death, the soul is immediately transferred to another human or even an animal. The way one lives on earth determines, as a reward or as a punishment, where one is transferred at the time of death.

Reincarnation is believed among some Westerners; Christianity condemns it. Orthodox Judaism believes that all dead souls are stored and will be liberated when the Messiah comes.

For Muslims, every step of their life and the time of their death has already been written. According to their belief, every Moslem has been assigned a predetermined mission on earth and he just has to find it. There is no possibility of refusing or escaping this mission. As a result, many Moslems feel that human interference with disease or death is irrelevant. Since their lives have already been scripted by fate, it is futile to try and alter destiny. What will be will be, and to attempt to take fate into human hands is presumptuous.

The experience of other cultures teaches us that there is more than one way to approach dying and death and should spur us to search for a better way.

Chapter 12

THE DIFFICULTY OF DEFINING
NATURAL DEATH IN HUMANS

Humans have no concept of natural death. They always interfere with it, and, in fact, make it so.

Only after describing how unnatural our current approach to death is, could we attempt a different approach to death and dying.

What is a natural death? Or, more to the point, why is human death so unnatural? By contrasting animal with human death, examining the notion of extended life and exploring the idea of a death instinct, we can better understand what a natural death is (and is not). What I hope to show you is that we interfere with the process of death to the extent that life ends in a completely artificial environment, and this is what makes death so difficult for most people.

OLD AGE IN ANIMALS

As I noted earlier, natural death in the wild is generally brutal and often occurs at the peak of maturity. Animals in the wild never die of a prolonged disease or old age. In contrast, domestic animals such as dogs or cats or any pet as well as animals in zoos live and die differently. Most often they receive medical care from veterinarians and have no problems acquiring food; predators are usually not a significant problem. Domesticated animals die in a way that is vaguely similar to humans (death in old age or after a prolonged disease). This is what I call a humanized death.

Sometimes we transfer the conditions of human death to animals, the assumption being that animals would certainly prefer the human way. In other words, animals would prefer old age and death after progressive incapacitation rather than the brutal death that is common in the wild. Of course, there is no rational basis for this assumption. To think a domestic animal is happy to be alive when weak, old and/or crippled is purely a human conceit. Nonetheless, societies for the prevention of cruelty to animals would probably disagree, believing that animals should die in an humane manner, not realizing the irony of that phrasing.

Animals are not familiar with nor have they evolved in old age the way humans have. Humans imposed this concept upon them. While animals have benefited from modern medicine through the use of various medications, it's conceivable that they don't desire old age and in fact would prefer to die earlier. It's conceivable because we know that when animals are put to sleep, they are neither conscious of life nor death. They do not know that they are dying because they do not know they are living. For them, all they want is to be without pain. For them to die or go to sleep is the same thing. They are not put to death; they are literally and figuratively just put to sleep.

Humans put animals to sleep out of kindness. Old dogs become blind, paralyzed, dislocate their hip joints and are difficult to feed. They become progressively inactive and even refuse to eat. It's possible that some owners put their pets to sleep because they find the animals have become a burden to them. Most veterinarians, however, suggest otherwise. Most pet owners take care of their animals in the most devoted manner for many years, and they put these pets to sleep not because of the imposition but out of concern and love for the animal. This is only fitting, since we have imposed old age on animals for our convenience and not because animals want it. What's thought provoking is that we do this kindness for animals but not for our fellow human beings.

It's also fascinating to realize that animals in the wild, unlike humans, enjoy perfect dentition (teeth) for almost their entire life. When the first flaw in a tooth occurs, they die shortly thereafter. The same is true for vision and hearing. Animals are designed to live only so long as all these functions operate perfectly; if they aren't operating perfectly, they quickly starve or are vulnerably to predators. Conditions are different for animals living in human contact. A great problem faced by veterinarians and animal keepers is that animals have all sorts of dental problems. But contrary to expectations, these problems aren't caused by what people feed animals or living conditions in zoos and laboratories. Dental problems arise because we have created old age for animals. In the wild, they don't live long enough for these problems to grow and spread. Humans, of course, develop problems with their teeth, eyes and other organs and survive for many years. Our bodies age and fall apart gradually, and aggressive medical treatment allows us to adapt and compensate for our failing system. Domesticated animals now enjoy the same treatment and slow dissipation. It's worth asking if we're doing the animals a kindness or causing them to suffer needlessly and unnaturally.

I strongly believe that in old animals there is what I call a death instinct. It is easy to observe old dogs or other old animals living in zoos. These animals are weak, inactive, and often handicapped. They sniff their surroundings much less, which is a serious handicap for animals since smell is their most important sense. They shy away from other individuals of the same species, they always run away when approached by an aggressive animal or offer no resistance. They have difficulty eating (teeth problems) and become emaciated or overeat and become overweight. Obesity is a serious problem in animals, much worse than in humans, because they have never been prepared for it from an evolutionary point of view. They walk awkwardly and prefer to stay still which aggravates the problem. Many other detailed observations caused me to conclude that old animals do not live the usual animal life as evidenced by their general appearance and behavior. A death instinct appears as soon as animals lack full maturity and strength or show any kind of irreversible handicap. For animals, a flawed life is no life at all, and that means death. To be alive but not be able to function at full strength is against their nature. They do not wish and would not know how to resist this death instinct if it was not for human intervention. They have no concept of death, and their natural response to infirmity is inactivity and sleep. To slip into a permanent sleep is no more alarming for a damaged animal than to slip into a temporary sleep.

What if we lived for 150 to 200 years? First, we would experience even more health problems than we do now as well as progressive mental deterioration. Invariably, we would become a burden to ourselves and other people. It's not just that we'd be a burden to our children, close relatives and friends, but great grandchildren would view us as nuisances without ever having known us when we were healthy and self-sufficient. We'd also become a major societal burden, straining the social security system beyond repair and draining off untold tax dollars for healthcare purposes. I've found that terminally ill patients frequently feel terrible guilt that they're imposing on others. This guilt would be exacerbated given an extended life. No one who has a deep attachment for his family and friends would want them to take care of him for 30, 40 or 50 years.

It's also important to consider how extended life might be nothing more than an extension of the boredom and uselessness many people feel after they retire. An additional 50 years of a meaningless existence isn't much of a gift. If you're too sick to work or if you've lost you're mental faculties or if you're viewed by society as non-functional, those additional years will be torture. It will make you hostile to the people who surround you and increase your wish to die sooner rather than later.

Extended life also isn't a solution for the current horror of dying and death. Living an additional 50 years doesn't mean that people will be more accepting of death when it comes. It simply means that the last tragic act will be postponed. No matter how many additional years extended life adds, it will never be enough to diminish our fear and anger as death approaches. That can only happen if we improve the quality of our death rather than the quantity of years we live. I have often met terminal patients who have started the process of dying. First, they were scared; then, they became used to it. To a proposal for some new treatment, their response is negative. The dying process is long and painful; I am well along the way now and I don't feel like starting all over at another date. I may as well finish now. In this case, the animal death instinct has resurfaced.

Jeanne Calment was a 123-year old-woman who lived in Arles, France. At the time of her death, she was the oldest person in the world with an official birth certificate. She had undergone numerous tests which found her sound in mind although she had quite a few handicaps. Imagine the world in which she lived in her final 20 years, a world in which not only had all her acquaintances died but also all her children. When asked during her last years of life how she saw her future, her answer was that it should be very short. Life was meaningless for her.

Still, it's likely that scientific breakthroughs will result in extended lives, and one has to wonder if this is unnatural. Psychologically and ethically, you could make a good case for it not being natural. If those additional years do nothing more than add life quantity at the expense of life quality, then there's something wrong with this concept. There has always been a generation gap. But when people are living in a world separated by three, four or more generations, the potential for conflict and animosity is huge.

Natural Death and Death Instinct

I suppose that dying of old age (or senescence) could be called natural death for humans only, because it is specific to and occurs only in humans. I would prefer to call this type of death a biological death, meaning the cells and organs of the body have reached a stage where they no longer function. Human death is more than biological, however, because we are aware of it. This is what makes it so difficult.

Indeed, in addition to being biological, human death (and only human death) is also a mental phenomenon. In humans, the death instinct is buried under deep layers represented by awareness and fear of death. Sigmund Freud speaks of a death instinct deeply buried in our mind and as real as our drive for survival. It surfaces under specific conditions when life is no longer bearable, as when one is aging or terminally ill. For instance, a terminally ill patient began to fall into a coma because of a fluid and electrolyte imbalance. In response to the patient's husband's request, I was intending to give her fluids intravenously which would extend her life for a few more days. When I asked her permission to start the intravenous line, her answer was, "If you want to." It was clear that the patient was prolonging her life for me (and her husband), not for herself. She really wanted to die, but she was willing to hang on for a few more days because I had made the request.

I do not think people in general and the medical profession in particular are aware of a death instinct in humans. They don't accept that people look forward to death. But I'm convinced that people do look forward to it when they cease to play a significant role in the world and their life becomes physically and emotionally unbearable. This system has been in place for all living species for billions of years. Toward the end of life, death can in some way be called natural. There is a call and appeal for it; it is registered within us; it is even fair to term it genetic.

Everyone can see this if one does not block it. Of course, when I mention this idea to the family, they usually become angry.

Humans Have to Define Their Own Approach to Death

It's not just the dying process that humans interfere with. We have a tendency to interfere with many different natural processes. In fact, if asked to define humans in comparison to other living creatures, I would answer without hesitation that what characterizes humans is their interference with natural processes. We are afraid to do it, pretend not to do it, do it hesitantly, awkwardly, and make many mistakes, but we do it all the time. Sometimes, we do it proudly and shamelessly.

Life has been evolving for billions of years and always has been regulated by natural selection and survival of the fittest, as described by Charles Darwin. With the appearance of Homo Sapiens, our unique consciousness—the awareness that we are alive and the ability to make choices independent of our biological drives—set us apart. Our hyperdeveloped brain enabled us to ignore biological law in certain instances. In animals, the brain is purely a biological instrument. In humans, it is also designed for consciousness and independent initiative.

In the animal kingdom, body and brain are in harmony because both are subject to the same biological laws. In humans, the independent mind tends to skip the biological laws although it is subject to them. At the time of death, the body receives this death as natural but the independent mind does not. This leads to the following paradox:

Natural death is normal, but human death is not.

What is a natural death for humans? How can we reconcile this paradox? We can start by stating that it's natural for humans during the aging process to fight and to be attracted to death at the same time. How much a person leans toward fighting it or moving toward it depends on age, health, associated disease, culture and individual personality. At the time of death, our mind refuses to accept death the way our body accepts it. It's consciousness and independent spirit makes this acceptance impossible. In fact, our minds revolt against death, and this revolt is what is natural. Even though our bodies go through the natural order of growth, maturity, senescence and death, our minds naturally resist the final stages.

Because we always interfere with the process of death, human death is man-made. Let us recognize that natural death does not exist and that we have to deal with this reality. Since there is no natural process of dying to rely on, we may as well courageously face it, deal with it, and make it.

We need to begin by defining what human death should not be. This supposes making a tabula rasa of the lies, hostility, fear, silence, physical suffering, isolation, taboos, and rituals that surround death. This is easier said than done, requiring both the dying individual and surrounding people to think in new ways about human death. It means everyone must be willing to explosure alternatives, be open to new ideas and be able to talk about their fears. Once these things take place, the dying person will be better able to express his wishes for a different and more meaningful way of dying. The following chapter will provide a fresh perspective on what death is, a perspective that will facilitate thinking about this subject in new ways.

Chapter 13

MIND, BODY AND THE NATURE OF DEATH

Cogito, ergo sum—I think, therefore I am. —Descartes

We cannot contemplate death without considering the different parts of us that die. When our bodies die, what happens to our minds, spirits and souls? Many philosophers and other experts have weighed in on this question. Modern quantum theory rejects the duality of mind and body; religious thinkers distinguish body and soul; philosophers clearly divide body and spirit; and there are classic thinkers such as Descartes who distinguish body and mind.

Without getting into a knotty philosophical debate, I'm going to talk about mind and body as separate entities for the purpose of this discussion. When you separate the mind from the body in the study of humans, you should never forget the basic difference between mind and body: Their different origins. The human body is the result of billions of years of animal inheritance and its biology is basically similar to that of all other animals. The mind is of very recent origin; it began to appear only a couple of million years ago and became fully formed only about 40,000 years ago with the Neanderthals. From an evolutionary point of view, the body appeared first, and it is only much later and very secondarily that the mind took root in it. Theilard de Chardin stresses that, although the body has little evolution left, the mind is still evolving.

As we'll see, these distinctions are crucial to how we approach death and dying and how we might change this approach.

Body as a Support for the Soul

Is the human body the proper support and carrier for our mind and soul? This isn't a silly or academic question; it has tremendous relevance to our perspective on death. If we were sure that the soul exists apart—if the body dies but the soul lives on—then it certainly would alleviate much of our fear of death. Of course, this issue becomes cloudy when we attempt to find the answer in the animal kingdom. If we take for granted that animals have no minds or souls, then their bodies certainly don't support and carry anything besides flesh, bones, organs and other bodily parts. Since we inherited our bodies from this animal world, it would stand to reason that bodies weren't designed for carrying the soul.

We've always questioned the purpose of our bodies; we've investigated it down to the cell's nucleus. We want to know not only how it works but why it sometimes doesn't work. Thus, it makes perfect sense to wonder if the body was created to carry our souls. We can question when we're young, but it becomes acute at the time of aging and death. The anxiety of death may be nothing more than a deficient body carrying a less deficient and more independent soul. Perhaps progress with the problem of death will be to find a more adequate body to carry the soul. Philosophers and thinkers (see The Thinker of Auguste Renoir) have always wondered about and pondered this question.

Some hold that body and soul are separate and regard the body with some contempt. This approach is seen in the Narrative by Plato on the death of Socrates and has been fully adopted by Christianity, which considers the body a burden to the soul. Religious authorities do not consider the body the proper receptacle for the soul and argue that the body makes too many biological demands (food, sex, etc.) that imperil the purity of the soul. Sexual abstinence, fasting, and even self-imposed physical suffering are three techniques used by religions to make the soul independent of the body. In fact, Christianity during the Middle Ages, justified burning a sinner or heretic alive as a way to free the soul from the defective body.

The argument about this issue has raged through the centuries. Aristotle didn't believe in separating the soul from the body and considered them as a total unit that could only artificially be looked at as two entities. Marcus Aurelius considered death a victory against the demands of our senses and the violence of our passions, the freedom of intelligence from its submission to the flesh.

From my perspective, it seems clear that the mind (or spirit or soul) is progressively and continuously increasing as we advance in age. We gain more experience and reason more often and better; our spiritual lives become deeper and enriched as we gain the reflective and meditative qualities that come with age. But as our minds and souls blossom, our bodies wither. A progressively improving mind within a progressively decaying body is a tragic development; at the very least it seems like a cruel one. Just as we reach a higher spiritual and mental plane, our bodies betray us. As we lay dying, this cruel joke makes us terribly sad.

DEATH OF THE BODY, DEATH OF THE MIND

Does the mind die? Does the soul and spirit? From a biological perspective, we can only say with authority that the body dies. As far as the mind is concerned, we consider it alive only because we are conscious of being alive. We really do not know if the mind (or spirit or soul) exists beyond consciousness. Death of the mind is not as obvious and does not occur the same way as death of the body. In fact, we really do not know how it occurs or even if it occurs. The mystery and uniqueness of human death is that it is more than cessation of biological life, more than death of the body. Brain death has become a common term, and it's widely accepted as the real measure of life's end; a complete cessation of consciousness signals the end according to many people's definitions of death even if the body keeps functioning. In this case, we become a vegetable; we function only biologically and not humanly.

There's been widespread debate on this subject in religious circles. Even in non-religious arenas, there's disagreement on whether the death of the mind should be considered the end (and the plug should be pulled) or if our lives are not over until our bodies say they are. Universal agreement on this issue would help still much of the acrimony that results when brain deaths occur but hearts beat on.

COORDINATION BETWEEN BODY AND SOUL DURING THE DYING PROCESS

The higher cerebral functions are mind, spirit, and soul. For our purposes here, let's define each of these functions (recognizing that these definitions are open to debate). Mind essentially refers to reason and logic. The spirit includes ethical and emotional values. The soul implies much higher values with some independence from the body. Certainly these terms overlap, but I'll use mind when referring to rationality, spirit when discussing ethics and soul when philosophy or religion are implied. What these three terms have in common is that they are specific to humans and are products of the hypertrophied human brain. These functions do not exist in animals, and this means that thinking in animals is subordinate to biological demands (hunger, thirst, etc.).

We understand biological or natural death as cessation of the body function. But how does death of the mind occur? Biology and medical books describe biological or natural death very well. It's unclear, however, how the mind dies. To assume that the mind has died when the brainwaves have disappeared is a faulty assumption because brainwaves can be present even when consciousness has temporarily or permanently disappeared. The way in which the mind, reflecting on itself and conscious of imminent death, reacts to the coming death, is poorly known. We do know that the mind is conscious of its own death, tortured by it and agonizes over it because it watches itself die. While the death of the human body might be a natural process, the death of the mind, soul and spirit is not; nature has made no provision for these intangible deaths.

The classic concept that our mind (or spirit or soul) is located in our brain is continuously challenged. No one really knows the exact site of the conscious (and unconscious) mind. Neurologists and neurosurgeons have studied the function of every anatomical site of the brain and have not been able to locate any site that could carry our mind. The exact location, if there is any, is a mystery. The perplexing question becomes: If our mind (or spirit or soul) has no anatomical existence, then what happens to it when we die? It is at the time of death that this mystery becomes acute and agonizing.

The classic concept is that body and soul are interdependent and that as body functions decrease with old age, so do mental functions. It is indeed a common observation that as people grow older and are less physically active, they experience diminished mental function. These aging people talk less, lose memory, do not recognize people and become more withdrawn. Many times, however, this parallel diminishment of mind and body doesn't occur.

I have seen people whose minds start to diminish first, with the disappearance of practically all mental functions while the body functions remain intact. This may be the result of senility, senile dementia, Alzheimer's disease, brain trauma or any other pathological condition associated with diminishing mental function characteristic of old age.

I have also seen the very opposite. Some people, up to their last breath, have an active and productive mind but their body organs (heart, lungs, kidneys, etc.) progressively fail. Their minds rebelliously refuse to die. There is nothing natural in this type of death; in fact it seems quite unnatural and even sadistic. When our minds are sharp and our bodies fail, death is difficult to accept. When our minds fail first or fail in tandem with our bodies, however, death is much more easily accepted.

Coordinating death of the body with that of the mind (or spirit and soul) is a problem we have yet to solve.

THREE REASONS WHY AGING IS NOT ALWAYS WHAT IT SEEMS

Natural evolution mandates that older generations must disappear to make room for younger ones. In the workplace, young people are often in a rush to take over. They've inherited this trait from our animal and human ancestry where young and physically strong individuals ruthlessly displaced and killed older ones. Physical capacities diminish and any job that requires physical stamina even to a slight degree may sometimes necessitate young replacement workers. Mental capacities also sometimes slow with age and the quick thinking required in the competitive business world may sometimes necessitate "fresh blood." While we can observe aging from physical and mental perspectives, we cannot always take what we observe for granted.

The first problem concerns a purely unsubstantiated extension of the biological laws (natural selection and survival of the fittest) to humans. Darwin (1859), the father of evolution, never said that the laws of evolution apply to the human species, although neodarwinian scientists desperately attempt to apply natural evolution to human evolution. The biological laws (birth, growth, maturity, reproduction, senescence, death, natural selection, survival of the fittest) apply to the human body the way they apply to the body of nonhuman creatures. The human mind may grossly go through some kind of cycle vaguely similar to the biological cycle, but this similarity is very superficial since the human mind was fully formed only 40,000 years ago. Nobody has yet satisfactorily described the evolution of the human mind (its appearance, growth, transmission from one generation to the next, senescence, and finally death).

The second problem involves the differences between biological evolution of the human body and evolution of the human mind which is completely novel in the evolutionary system. The transmission of body characteristics from one generation to the next is essentially genetic in nature, while the transmission of mental values is essentially cultural. In the human world, the new generation has much to learn from the older one, while in the animal world there is no such thing or at least very little. In fact, my definition of humanity is the ability to transmit values culturally as well as genetically, while in the animal and plant kingdoms the transmission is almost exclusively genetic.

Third, the concept that the older generation has to make room for the new one may sound logical from a Darwinian perspective but from a human point of view it does not make any sense. Old age in humans has established its own identity and separate life during evolution. Most young people don't have genocidal impulses toward senior citizens. The human mind may have a life cycle of its own and may not show any sign of senescence regardless of advanced age. This reinforces the fact that death of the human body may be natural, but the death of the human mind is still an unresolved issue.

To those who claim that death of the human mind is natural, consider that thinking man tries to escape the laws of natural death and hangs on even after the biological functions of the body start to disappear. The sad conclusion is that the human mind, although witnessing the cessation of all biological functions, does not want to disappear and therefore is at variance with nature.

On one side, we have the spectacle of a body progressively aging and dying of senescence or diseases of increasing severity. Senescence of the human body occurs in a very disorganized way. Some organs start to decline first and may even reach an advanced state of malfunction while other organs remain intact, making human death more cruel as the different organs fail one after the other.

On the other side, the mind does not want to die, does not know how to die and yet is conscious of dying in some atrocious way because it sees the body disintegrating and dying.

This is not a simple and natural process. "Quos vult perdere Jupiter dementat," means that nature punishes man for his consciousness by making him insane at the time of dying and death. What's frightening is that we have to handle this insane stage by ourselves without help from nature or any divinity.

Given this scenario, animals might be considered lucky to die the way in which they do. Lacking a soul, spirit or mind (though there are religions that might debate this point), animals can be considered to die peacefully, even though violently. Some people often achieve this peaceful death because their minds have degenerated to the point that they're not conscious of their dying. They aren't tortured by their minds instinctively striving to interpret and solve the inscrutable, unsolvable problem of their deaths.

We always have questioned any mechanisms given to us by nature and always have attempted to understand, revise, and modify them. We eventually have to determine our own mechanism of death, regardless of whether it belongs to or is different from any plan of nature or of any tradition. We need to use our ability to meditate and ponder the problem of death. This endeavor will require a dynamic approach to the medical, psychological, philosophical, and metaphysical basics that form human culture.

Later on, I'll suggest the elements that might comprise this approach.

CHAPTER 14

TREATING DEATH AS A TRANSITION

"The past is like a funeral gone by, the future comes like an unwelcome guest" —Edmund Gosse

To suggest a new approach to death may sound like a violation of the natural order of things. Death is what it is, and to attempt to transmute it into something else is wrong—so the traditionalists might say. Others might fight the notion of a new approach to be laughable. How in the world can you change the way a society deals with death? People are naturally going to fight against it and want healthcare professionals to assist them in this fight.

I'd like to suggest an alternative point of view. Before doing so, however, I need to disabuse you of the idea that our current mode of death is natural; that to rebel against it is to rebel against natural laws. In reality, human death has become an extraordinarily unnatural process.

SURVIVAL OF THE FITTEST AND OTHER BARBARIC CONCEPTS

Over time, the human race has moved further and further away from the Darwinian principles of natural selection and survival of the fittest. In fact, you could summarize the history of mankind as follows: A continuous, desperate and often unsuccessful attempt to become free of the laws of nature and natural evolution. This is not to say that everyone throughout history would agree with this summary. Bismarck, the German chancellor at the end of the nineteenth century, maintained that wars were necessary to "purify" the human race and to dispose of the excess. Nazi Germany wanted to purify the human race by eliminating the misfits. They might subscribe to the concept of natural selection and view death as a means to a glorious end.

But most people—at least most people with a strong sense of morality and humanity—would find nothing natural about human death.

Medicine, certainly, is a tool to delay the natural process of aging and to postpone the natural death for as long as possible. In a broader context, people have always tried to strike some sort of accommodation between natural laws and human laws. The wearing of shoes or clothing (nature would mandate thick or hairy skin) and inventing fire against rigorous climates (nature would rather select a species adapted to cold or to hunger) are just two examples of how we have circumvented natural laws. Other examples include storage of food or building habitats, care of the weak, widows, and orphans, charity, love, religion, the rise of Christianity among Roman slaves, the passive resistance of Ghandi against British imperialism and fighting starvation in Somalia and genocide in Bosnia. None of this has anything to do with the laws of natural evolution.

The same is true for medical care and care of the elderly. Natural law would dictate that: No one is allowed to be sick and no one is allowed to become old. At the slightest sign of any disease or the slightest appearance of aging, the individual would be ruthlessly eliminated. This is how nature has worked for millions of years and perfected the living species. Nature does not give a hoot about ethics or the value of the elderly to society.

In the beginning this is how human nature worked, but later this is not how human culture wanted it to work. Not so long ago, the average life span was forty years of age and the whole population was relatively healthy because no one had the means or the knowledge to handle the sick and the old. Very few were sick or old for too long because very few could stay alive under those conditions. Today (outside of third world countries) the average life span has practically doubled, since an average citizen who uses ordinary available care could easily reach the age of eighty and beyond and still be in relatively good health. People live longer and are healthier not because the best individuals are selected for survival (this is how nature works) but because of our concern for each other and the care available for the sick and elderly (this is how human culture works). Keeping in good health and extending life certainly is a tremendous achievement against the laws of nature. At the same time, however, extending life brings its own problems, as I've discussed throughout the book. What it comes down to is that there are three available modes of death, one that might be considered natural and two that might be considered unnatural. Let's briefly define each of these modes:

1. Brutal death. This has been handed down from our animal ancestry and involves a violent and painful end. An atavistic mode of death, this is the one humans simultaneously rebel against and perfect. While no one wants to die suddenly and at the hands of a predator, we also persist in perfecting weapons (from nuclear bombs to handguns) that make it more likely that this will be our fate.

2. Extended aging or disease. This slow, painful death is the result of modern technology and medicine, and it is the most common form and the most agonizing from emotional and physical standpoints.

3. Future natural death. This is the mode that is being discussed and debated now, though it has not been embraced or implemented by many. It assumes the use of pharmacological drugs when death becomes inevitable. It also is responsible for the trend of various institutions allowing people to choose their method of dying and even their time of death, at least when they reach a terminal stage. Tremendous progress in pharmacological drugs make death possible in a relaxed and completely painless way, and it puts control of the process in the hands of those who are dying. Rather than let death follow its inevitable course, this future natural death would be regulated and directed with pharmacological drugs. This method does not necessarily make death come sooner, but it certainly makes it less painful and more peaceful. I will expand on the last mode of death in the following chapters.

How Life is Terminated Today

We have become increasingly involved in extending life in the elderly and fighting death in terminally ill patients by all available scientific means rather than letting the sick and elderly die. This approach has become so routine that we forget to ask its purpose. Almost every time I am involved in the management of a terminally ill patient or an elderly patient with advanced physical and mental handicaps, family members find a way to ask: How long is the patient going to live; when is he going to die; and how long will he receive life support treatment? Sometimes the dying patient asks these questions. Whenever I start talking about pulling the plug , they usually protest that they do not want to precipitate death and want it to be natural. But I can see in their faces that if I were to take the responsibility for pulling the plug, they wouldn't oppose the decision.

Still, they become stuck on the issue of natural death and decide to fight it to the end. In the name of natural death, we are fighting for something that is essentially meaningless. We are stuck with a system of extending life and dying which is based on customs, misunderstandings, taboos, obsolete concepts and fear of death. The collusion of healthcare professionals, family members and the dying to preserve this system is nothing less than collective insanity.

Certainly some people escape this insanity, live long, healthy lives and die relatively peacefully (usually in their sleep). But the majority suffer through prolonged illnesses and a gradual, agonizing descent into death. Even more insidious, a fear of being artificially kept alive and plunging into this nightmarish death is the main source of anxiety in people's final days, weeks or months.

This fear is maintained and even magnified as we age, and when we reach the end stage of life we all are compelled to fight death with every possible means. While this fear might be repressed by healthy people, it surfaces in the sick and elderly.

ACKNOWLEDGING A TRANSITION WE'VE BEEN MAKING FOREVER

Dying is a transition between life and death. Like all major changes, it's frightening. But it's also a change that can be facilitated. Thinking about it this way helps us get past our fear of tampering with nature. We understand the need to seek help when going through other changes in our lives—divorce, losing a job and so on. This is another transition that we can make easier and less painful.

Untreated, this transition does tremendous damage, but it's one that we can treat pharmacologically; the intervention for human death is not to fight against or prevent death but simply to focus on its abnormal aspect. If we implement this approach, we will not only improve the quality of our deaths but the quality of our lives. Most of us don't really deal with the prospect of our deaths until we're on the brink of dying. It's too frightening to do so earlier, and so we leave it to the end of our lives. If you visit a home for senior citizens, you'll often find elderly people sitting alone in wheelchairs with sad, pensive expressions. Talk to them, and if they're honest they'll tell you they're thinking about death. They're doing so individually and in isolation; there's little or no group or even one-on-one discussion. It's a private matter.

In fact, it should be public. If it were more out in the open and if there were more resources to deal with it, we wouldn't die in terrible isolation. We know that when the patient becomes terminal, the earlier treatment is started, the more effective it is. When treatment is initiated much later because too much time is spent fighting death, the fear of death takes root in the human psyche and is difficult to reverse. There is little education or preparation for death, although it is desperately needed for the dying as well as the living. It is only by seeing more people dying peacefully and without fear that we will learn to live and die peacefully and without fear. As we see more people dying in fear and anxiety, we accept this as natural and don't look for other options.

This vicious cycle needs to be addressed, and it needs to be addressed in the way we would approach any disease. More study, research, statistical data, and clinical investigation are necessary to test and improve new approaches to dying and death. Access to the latest information has to be developed and this knowledge, although available in a few publications, is barely known (Choice In Dying, The Chalice of Repose Project, Wisconsin Cancer Pain Initiative) and specialized consultations will be needed. We know more can be done for a patient with widespread cancer than chemotherapy which often produces only temporary remission. This does not mean that chemotherapy or other medical treatments should be neglected. But other considerations which are more necessary as the patient approaches the terminal stage also should come into play.

There is nothing sacred about the transitiion between life and death. Contrary to what some people believe, it can and should be interfered with rather than pursue its natural course. Our present mode of death is man-made and abnormal. Transitional traits can be divided into two groups: physical and emotional. The physical characteristics consist of physical pain and debilitation. The emotional components are multiple and can be placed under the heading of depression and other related feelings such as anxiety, apprehension, fear and so on.

Any non-dying patient can present various combinations of these traits and usually get the proper treatment for them. When presented by a dying patient, however, these traits are barely recognized or treated because we consider it as natural and do not recognize that this transitional condition calls for a specific diagnosis and treatment. In a dying patient we let these symptoms become progressive as death nears. We accept the fact that there is no hope for a cure for dying, and even if there was hope for a cure in the beginning, it eventually disappears. Everyone is convinced that there is no way out and all one sees in the future is a progressive worsening of all the symptoms, physical pain, debilitation, depression, and anxiety. Increasing hopelessness is a sure sign that this transitional condition is being ignored.

By acknowledging this transitional state, however, we can approach it calmly and peacefully (even ecstatically). If the physical pain and depression/anxiety can be thoroughly addressed, the fight against death can be replaced by receiving death.

The transition from life to death afflicts the healthy as well as the sick; the dread of this transition is present in everyone's mind well before the time of dying. Even if we try not to think about it when we're young and healthy, the fear roils about just below the conscious level. By middle age it breaks through to a conscious level and in old age dominates our thoughts. If we can bring this transition into the open, recognize it easily, describe it fully, and treat it vigorously without interfering with any other medical treatment, we will come that much closer to turning dying and death into a natural process.

Here's what's unnatural about dying and death: To be deprived of the experience of death when we are capable of facing it; to be forced into an experience of death that is not of our choosing. What's natural is to receive or at least to accept death; to conquer it does not mean fight it. Since we cannot avoid it, why not die under the most favorable circumstances and in a situation of our own choosing? Since man is subjected to evolution and even revolution, why not use these to select and create a mode of death that would alleviate fear, anxiety, pain, concern, guilt? Many people have lived a normal or even fantastic life, only to have it spoiled by an abnormal death. Endings don't have to be tragic and sully all that has come before.

There is such a thing as proper education and preparation for dying. It would be ideal if old people, who are retired from an active life familiarized themselves and all others around them with the concept of death, even when they are completely healthy. By talking about, thinking about and preparing for death, they might shorten and soften the painful parts of it. We will no longer say, "He fought or lost the battle against death." We will say instead: "He was well prepared to die" or "He died peacefully."

This is as opposed to making heroes out of people who fight death. The media reports stories about people who have fought a spreading cancer to the bitter end and they are glorified for fighting. These stories make death appear as a bitter enemy armed with its own weapons against whom we are engaged in a deadly duel; there's a bizarre quixotic tone to these battles, as if it were noble to dream the impossible dream of beating death. In almost every instance, this noble fight description comes from those who surround the dying person rather than the dying person himself. It may assuage the living to describe a loved one in this manner, but it provides no solace or satisfaction for most people who are dying. The real victory in this battle is for the dying person is to make peace with and receive death. The real defeat is to continuously reject and fight death.

I always have been leery of stoic terminal patients who insist on dying as heroes or martyrs and refuse all sedation in order to maintain that image to the very end. The danger and the underlying purpose of this stoic behavior is to make others feel guilty. It communicates to them that death is dreadful and enormous courage must be summoned to face it. The more a loved one suffers because of this martyrdom, the more guilty everyone feels. It is undeserved guilt; no one is forcing a dying person to suffer.

How different it would be if the patient died at home surrounded by family, even if death occurred a few hours or days earlier. Fortunately, more and more people are choosing this and other alternatives to the norm. Doctors are well aware that an increasing number of patients and their families are resisting treatment that extends the quantity of life at the cost of quality.

Unfortunately, the medical profession isn't leading this resistance. They have a tendency to remain neutral and follow tradition when treating others, but they are likely to join the resistance when they are diagnosed with a terminal disease, refusing to subject themselves to the treatments they impose on others.

A New Specialty to Treat a New Condition

Although it is not a medical problem, the medical profession always has considered it a medical decision to let or not to let a patient die. Laboring under a conservative mindset, many doctors believe that there is no right-to-die under any circumstance. The patient and family, unprepared for and terrified of death, accept the medical decision because they are glad to let someone else who seems more knowledgeable make this decision.

Thanatology (a complex word of Greek origin, which means science of death) tries to address the issue. This science is never taught to doctors, nurses, religious ministers or social workers. Thanatology is a morbid word and a contradiction, since science is the study of life and not death. If science must deal with the issue of death in a terminal patient, it does so solely to avoid it. All this makes it understandable why the mechanism of death is poorly understood by professionals as well as everyone else. How the different systems of the mind and body integrate with each other to keep us alive and how they dis-integrate at the time of death is a subject rarely investigated. How our conscious and unconscious mind reacts to dying remains a scientific mystery. Psychiatrists and psychologists have demonstrated that when a patient reaches a terminal stage due to an irreversible disease, the concept of death is definitely registered in the patient's mind. The relationship of death to consciousness and unconsciousness, however, is of little interest to scientists.

Psychologists and psychiatrists are more concerned with the following question:

If the coming death is known but buried in the unconscious mind of a terminally ill patient, is it best to make the patient fully conscious of it and discuss it openly or should the patient be allowed to die without ever being fully conscious of the coming death?

It's difficult to answer this question because some patients are better off knowing while others are not. I have given some peace of mind to many dying patients just by telling them they would die soon. Although they strongly suspected it and may have known it for certain, the fact that a doctor was confirming this fact allowed them to make important decisions about treatment from a truly informed perspective. Conversely, I have treated just as many dying patients to whom I said nothing because they never asked or the family objected. How to know who should be informed and who should not—not to mention how and when they should be informed—are crucial issues that need to be addressed.

It's also important that dying patients have a friend or family member with whom they can talk about these issues. I've had a number of patients aware that they were going to die soon but didn't have anyone with whom they felt comfortable talking about it. Equally troubling is when dying patients are surrounded by people who interfere with patients who are trying to come to terms with their approaching deaths; they interfere by projecting their attitudes about death, whether they do or do not want to know everything. Either attitude is fine provided it is not imposed on others. What I find odd is that psychologists, social workers and even some psychiatrists who have no experience dealing with dying patients are called in and suddenly act as if they were authorities on the subject of dying. They invariably do more harm than good, projecting their own fears and ignorance and making patients even more confused and anxious than they already are. They attempt to impose their ideas although they never dealt with a dying patient in their career; they often step forward and presume to be an authority on this matter. All they do is project their own concept or fear of death and confuse the issue.

Near Death Experience (NDE) is another area that deserves more study and research. An increasing number of people are reporting NDEs, and it seems that everyone might benefit if science looked at these experiences with an objective rather than a dismissive eye. We might learn something that could better prepare people for the end of their lives.

All of these issues compels us to take Thanatology seriously. Or at the very least, we should acknowledge that dying is a disease that demands scientists and scientific discipline to investigate it. What I'm suggesting is very much different than emergency medicine, the function of which is to ignore and fight death at all costs or gerontology, which is the science of keeping aging people alive as long as possible under any condition. A new specialty should focus on the dying process and management of the dying patient rather than pushing death away. Not all doctors, surrounding families or dying patients will accept this new area of specialization, but many will recognize its value. Specialists in treating the transition between life and death will help eliminate the hysteria that marks the end of many lives, and they will even collaborate with the patient (who they may or may not "know") to provide for specific needs. One person may desire to stop certain medical procedures; another might want different or more extensive procedures. The goal is to treat dying patients to help them with their transition rather than fight death. This is much more than a semantic difference, and it means that doctors who specialize in treating living patients will have to step aside (or become trained in treating this transitional condition).

Chapter 15

DRUG THERAPY:
THE MEANS TO ACHIEVE A BETTER DEATH

Primum non nocere: First, do no harm. —Hippocrates

Throughout our history, people have readily accepted the system of dying proposed by tradition, religion, witchcraft and medicine. Unprepared for death, we quickly gravitate to whatever system is in vogue. Our irrational fear of death drives us toward whatever process is available.

Because of recent advances in pharmacology and related medical applications, a new process is possible. It could revolutionize our approach to both death and life and deal more effectively with our fear than anything in the past. To understand what these pharmacological advances might mean, we need to first look at them within the context of the following three questions:

1. Why is it so difficult for many people to give up traditional approaches?

2. What traditional or inherited approaches should be kept?

3. What are the most promising future approaches that should be studied and tested?

REFUSING TO BE BOUND BY TRADITION

It's fair to wonder whether the current system of death is so entrenched that it would be virtually impossible to initiate any type of reform, let alone a revolution. Let's consider whether any type of significant change is really possible.

From the standpoint of dissatisfaction with the present system, it certainly seems that people would be receptive to an alternative. No matter how people die today, they and their loved ones complain about it. There are always complaints about doctors who do too much and too little; about how much someone is suffering; about unnecessary procedures and rude or ignorant treatment by nurses. You would think that this widespread dissatisfaction would make improvement easy. Not so. The French poet Boileau said: "<u>La critique est aisee, mais l'art est difficile</u>—Criticism is easy but art is difficult."

Unfortunately, once a system is established and organized, it gets its strength from the establishers. People with vested interests in the current system—healthcare administrators and professional staff, insurance companies and others—see no reason to make changes that might decrease their power and income. Stagnation is the curse of mankind. Besides, people disagree on what should replace the old system and recognize that the transition to any new system would be difficult. The French writer de Saint-Exupéry (1950) said it very well: "*Il n'y a pas d'ascention sans lutte contre la pesanteur*—One cannot ascend without fighting gravity."

In my own practice, I have attempted to improve the way in which patients under my care die, and I believe I have done so successfully. To make the changes I have made in my approach, however, required a radical shift in my perception and a willingness to break from medical tradition.

What has helped me make this break—and what might help you— is recognizing that there is no absolute or divine way of approaching death. Yes, each individual comes from a different background and brings a different perspective to dying. But no one should feel as if they need to conform to a given custom or religion based on his or her background if it makes dying difficult. Everyone should realize that his or her choice about how to die should be dictated by the best way to find relief from emotional or physical pain, regardless of previous beliefs. Willingness to free oneself from tradition can make dying a positive experience. I am convinced that dying under the proper circumstances and at the proper time can take much of the fear and pain out of the process.

We need to understand and accept that our present mode of dying is man-made rather than God-given. Though people will certainly use religious arguments to hold onto old practices, they are defending a system inspired and designed by man. It helps to look a death from a historical perspective to realize how fragile tradition is. As I've demonstrated throughout this book, different cultures, religions and eras all have viewed dying and death differently. What made perfect sense to one group of people seems like insanity to another. While certain people throughout history were glad to die because they were certain there was an afterlife waiting for them, others believe this life is all there is and therefore resist death with all their might.

Many people, unfortunately, lack this historical perspective and resist any change to tradition. They don't understand that nothing is static in life and evolutionary changes are the very definition of life. The hostility that one meets when change is proposed just means that one has to keep trying to find different ways to foster change, not that one must give up. My favorite expression is we are traditional by nature and revolutionary by culture. Our approach to death is determined by the history of a specific culture. There is nothing absolute or final in any of these approaches. What is the rule today will be the exception tomorrow. This fact should give us the courage to challenge traditions that are no longer viable.

WHAT IS TO BE KEPT OF THE TRADITIONAL APPROACHES

Just as we need to let go of certain traditions, we need to identify others that are still useful and keep or modify them. For instance, we can learn a great deal from the serenity and ceremony of acceptance that characterized our approach to death more than 200 years ago and that still is maintained by certain Asian cultures. There is comfort in tradition, and to rob dying people of all that they know—of all their customs and practices—isn't the right answer either. A combination of the new and the old is a sensible strategy.

Doctors certainly could benefit from a better acquaintance with traditional approaches. For instance, humility and serenity were two traits that dominated our thoughts and actions about death in the past. Although scientific thinking is necessary for satisfactory management of a sick patient, one has to understand that death is irrational, resistant to any natural or philosophical explanation. Modern man is often instinctively rational, but sometimes death has to be approached in a non-rational way. This means that doctors shouldn't always face death behind a mask of scientific reason and authority. It makes more sense for the physician to be humble in dealing with a disease he never cures.

I'm not implying that doctors should simply shrug their shoulders and say, There's nothing I can do. What I'm suggesting is that there should be more empathy and less scientific reason and objectivity. In a way, doctors have a more important role to play in this process because ministers, rabbis and other religious figures often are absent from the bedsides of dying patients. By default, doctors are the only ones available to assume this new and often uncomfortable role.

It's sad to admit that not all doctors are willing to assume it. Many times I have seen patients ready to discuss their coming death with the doctor, and the doctor walks away using some excuse, unable to admit to either the patient or himself that he is terrified of taking on this quasi-religious role. If, for whatever reason, the doctor cannot deal with death and the dying, he should admit this to himself, to the family of his patient and even to the patient. The worst thing he can do is ignore the person who is dying.

There are certain traditional doctor-patient relationships worth maintaining that doctors have moved away from. Years ago, family doctors often were valuable replacements for religious figures when people were dying. They were close to the patient and the patient's family, and they were willing and able to talk to dying people about the issues that concerned them. Today, doctors often don't help their patients accept death but help them fight it to the bitter end. To a certain extent, doctors haven't embraced this approach as much as it's been thrust upon them by society, hospitals and families of the dying person. Gone are the times when the family doctor held the hand of the dying patient, sharing the pain and anguish of the patient as well as the family's sorrow. He was part of the solemnity that became evident as death approached, and his sadness could not be distinguished from that of the surrounding people. This touching scene has been immortalized in paintings by famous artists such as Edvard Munch.

The modern physician today (especially young specialists) becomes virtually hyperactive in the face of death, proposing one procedure after another to keep the patient alive and becoming more agitated as death gets closer. He is anxious and frenetic as opposed to the calm family doctor of the past. Ironically, the modern doctor does not believe the patient is dying naturally, but that he is indirectly killing him because all the medical equipment at his disposal cannot manage to keep him alive. As death nears, he feels diminished, frustrated and humiliated. When the patient finally dies, he berates himself and wonders what he could have done to prevent the final outcome. He is angry at everyone, including the dead patient and himself.

If I exaggerate this state of mind a bit, it's only to make the contrast between the modern approach and the traditional one crystal clear. The calm and humility that family doctors possessed is something that might serve doctors well now and in the future.

Rationale for Implementing a New Drug Regimen for Terminal Patients

We are burdened with concepts about death and dying that are a reaction against animal death and a result of our acute human awareness that we're dying. Add to this mix the notion that we should extend life past a rational point and the fact that we're more attached to life than ever before. All this has become ingrained, and it's difficult for us to see alternatives.

But there are alternatives, and we can see them if we accept that all these things have been imposed on us in one way or another and are neither natural nor immutable. Man is free to accept or reject any part of his cultural environment and to determine his approach to life and death according to his interest. Of course, this is more of a goal than a reality; I'm describing a pathway on which we are struggling along. We are entitled to study the past and present history of the various approaches to death, to evaluate what is scientifically available in terms of medical progress and determine what is our best choice for life.

Right now the choices we've been making about dying and death are tragic. But I'm tremendously optimistic that humans are sufficiently adaptable to make wise choices. We now possess the knowledge and scientific means to ease the tension and anxiety associated with dying and death—not only for the dying person but for the family as well. A terribly negative experience can be transformed into a positive one for many of us.

To do so requires changes in the way we approach death. This approach may not be for everyone and may be applicable only for certain people under certain conditions. It is mostly for terminal patients suffering physical pain, fear, and anxiety and for their suffering families. This may not be the ideal strategy but it strikes me as a vast improvement over what we presently embrace.

Using drugs to ease people's suffering may strike some critics as artificial interference. From a big picture perspective, this argument against pharmacological drugs is absurd, given how we constantly interfere with and modify the natural order of things in all aspects of our life. From a medical perspective, this intervention is no more unnatural than the way in which we extend life through extraordinary measures. In fact, the use of drugs to ease pain and suffering and foster an acceptance of death seems one of the most natural human reactions I can imagine. After all, we've developed these wonderful drugs that we know would be effective for both the dying patient and surrounding family; we know they desperately crave relief from their fear and pain. Our ingenuity in solving problems through science is a remarkably human trait, and it's one that we could put to use to solve the problem of how we die.

I'm not underestimating the obstacles to doing so; I understand that it takes a certain amount of courage to broach the subject of drug management with dying patients and their families; and I admit drug management is not for everyone. Still, combined with an ecstatic and positive mindset as death approaches (similar to what people report during Near Death Experiences), this drug management concept makes eminent sense for many people.

If we are to manage the dying process through drug therapy, we need to acknowledge the relationship between the two types of pain terminal patients experience. For instance, a cancer patient is suffering due to the growth and spread of the tumor itself. But the patient is also suffering because of depression, despair and confusion about his condition. Though these two types of pain are independent of each other in one sense, in another they're inextricably linked. A negative synergy arises, and as each type of pain exacerbates the other, the sum of the suffering grows.

Most caregivers are unable or unwilling to treat these two types of pain as linked and don't deal with the physical and emotional problems simultaneously. The physician in charge of treating the physical symptoms treats only the physical pain, and the physician in charge of treating the emotional symptoms (which is done much less frequently) treats only the emotional pain. Medications for treating one type of pain have nothing to do with the medications for treating another type. Although the symptoms may overlap and even be similar, the medications operate independently. One type of complaint may need analgesia, surgery, radiotherapy or chemotherapy and another type may need antidepressants, anxiolytic drugs or psychotherapy. Unfortunately what happens most often is that the two caregivers (the treating physician and a psychiatrist, for instance) barely communicate, and the patient is not treated holistically.

As a result, the patient usually still suffers a significant amount of physical and emotional pain. This leads to both doctors and patients doubting the efficacy of their treatment. Sometimes the treatment is withdrawn because of this doubt, and patients and doctors often come to believe that it's normal to suffer emotionally and physically when dying. This belief leads them to think that any type of interference in this natural process is wrong. Such a belief may seem absurd at first glance, but it's one that consciously or not infects the attitudes of healthcare practitioners and patients alike.

To counter this belief and allow ourselves to consider a drug management alternative, we need to understand the three key treatment areas when dealing with terminal patients.

First, there's physical pain. This can involve any pain associated with spread of a malignancy, such as malignant metastasis to bones, nerve compression, compression of a vital organ and so on. About one third of terminal patients have some kind of pain during the last few weeks or even months preceding death. Too often, doctors undertreat patients with physical pain and at times even ignore it.

Anxiety and depression is the second area. Most patients, perhaps 80%, are aware of the coming death. Almost half of these patients, however, don't talk about it and often give the impression they're unaware that death is imminent. My experience has convinced me that almost all dying patients, at some level of the conscious or unconscious mind, have become aware that they are dying or at least feel that something is seriously wrong and are apprehensive and fearful about it. Most patients express some anxiety about death at least once during the dying process. Most doctors ignore when patients articulate their fears, even when they clearly are terrified.

Before moving on to the third area, I should interject that if the physical pain, depression and anxiety associated with imminent death can be relieved through medication, the dying process would not be nearly so horrific. I should also add that as much sense as this statement might make, putting it into practice is another issue entirely.

The third area we need to consider is the attitude of caregivers. Assuming the physical and emotional pain is under control, most people achieve a greater acceptance of dying than is commonly believed. If patients wish to speak about their coming deaths, doctors need to be open to this discussion and not attempt to sidetrack it or ignore it. They should also respect the patient who spends his last days, weeks or months in an ecstatic state rather than view it with alarm, repulsion or as if the patient has taken leave of his senses. In other instances, patients will wish not to talk about their fears and feelings related to death, and doctors should again respect this attitude and not force patients to talk about it.

To determine a therapeutic regimen for a dying patient, these three areas need to be addressed. Certainly there can be overlap between the areas and the lines dividing them are somewhat arbitrary, but they help us look at the process holistically. Looking at it this way makes it easier to see that there is an interconnectedness that doctors, patients and their families frequently ignore. We need to move past our traditional, narrow ways of treating and perceiving death and explore other options. While we're never going to eliminate awareness of death, we can become more receptive to it. We now possess the technology, medications and counseling expertise to make dying and death a positive and even ecstatic experience. The array of drugs available aren't perfect, and they may need to be tinkered with and tailored to individual conditions and concerns. But they need to be used more aggressively and innovatively. At the moment, we have only used them hesitantly and experimentally.

The action of all these drugs is well known to medical professionals—internists, anesthesiologists, pharmacologists, and psychiatrists specialized in psychopharmacology. Some of these professionals have compiled a long list of available medications and even recommended the use of some specific ones for the management of selected patients at the terminal stage. What is now needed is a very flexible, organized regimen for widespread use in patients with generalized cancer or any other terminal disease. In general, doctors are secretive about the use of these drugs and prescribe them only in limited quantity at the very end stage when the family starts to scream louder and louder, "Doctor, do something!" It is only at the end that the caring physician finally understands the meaning of the sentence, "Doctor, do something." Up until this point, he has been blinded by his role as lifesaver, life preserver and even lifegiver. He does not understand that the integrity of life demands a happy end. When death becomes evident, one should not become blind to it but attempt to face it clear-eyed and reduce the physical and emotional suffering as much as possible.

Today, we live in what I call a medication era. The amount of prescribed medication is staggering. I know people who practically live on drugs and take stimulants in the morning, sedatives at night and various vitamins and minerals during the day. I am aware of many patients who abuse hormones. It is unbelievable how frequently doctors prescribe antibiotics preventively, risking allergic reactions and ultimately rendering these antibiotics ineffective.

Yet when it comes to prescribing medications to a dying patient, one who will not be harmed by any long-term effect, the systematic prescription of medication for physical pain, depression, and anxiety is infrequent and even rare. The medications given are almost always too little and too late, for fear that they may interfere with the pseudo-heroic measures the doctor is taking to extend the patient's life.

Selection of Patients for Drug Treatment

It's ironic that the medications to relieve depression and anxiety, often denied to terminal patients, are rather generously prescribed to relieve the very same symptoms in the surrounding family. Widows and soon-to-be widows (more than widowers) frequently take some medication. It is bizarre that the risk of drug addiction and long-term negative effects are barely considered for the surrounding family but often are a concern for the dying patient.

What I recommend is not just more medication for those who are dying but a completely new approach to terminal patients. First, we should broaden the list of those we consider terminal beyond those with incurable cancer to include people with failing vital organs such as the heart, kidneys, liver, and lungs. We should also include very elderly people with multiple medical problems who have reached the terminal stage of life and who specifically express no interest in staying alive. Anyone disinterested in the artificial prolongation of their lives should be classified as terminal.

This definition isn't easy for doctors or family members to accept. The former group is angry at the dying for refusing to respond to life-saving therapies and the latter is angry because they don't appreciate all that's being done for them. As a result, it's very hard for anyone to broaden the definition of terminal. Our impulse is to narrow it further.

The dying themselves are weakened by their condition and unable to stand up for their rights and demand to be included in the terminal group. Instead, they often become the receptacle of all our frustrations, including our fear of death. Terminal people feel deep inside that we resent them because they have activated and brought to the surface our unconscious fear of death. What terminal people observe is that we the living are interested in relieving our fear of death rather than helping them deal with their own fear of death. When the immediate members of a family surrounding a dying person take sedatives, it is to relieve their anxiety as they watch their relative die, while sometimes they and the treating doctors do less to deal with the pain, fear, anxiety and depression of the dying.

What I am proposing is simply an early and aggressive regimen of medication to improve the physical and mental condition of the dying patient. The regimen should be put in motion only at the specific request of a well-informed patient and with the consent of the family. It is possible that some terminal patients will not need it. Or it may be that they don't need it at first but do need it later. Flexibility is important, and doctors and family members should monitor both the mental and physical condition of patients to determine what medications are needed at different points in time.

Reason for Undertreatment of Dying Patients

Doctors overlook new drugs that can make dying and death painless, that can relieve depression or anxiety, and that can even produce euphoria. Because these drugs can make dying bearable, I don't understand why they are not used in a more generalized way and upon request. The objections to using these drugs for dying patients remind me of the objections of sedating women in labor during the previous century. People objected to sedation based on the belief that God intended women to "labor in sorrow," and also on the fear that excessive sedation might make spontaneous breathing of the newborn more difficult. Terminal patients should not labor in sorrow as they're dying nor should they be denied excessive sedation.

Certainly some medications are used to relieve the distress of dying patients today, but they are used insufficiently and in a haphazard, hesitant, and even embarrassing manner. It is time to use them openly and rationally as well as to organize and codify their use for dying patients. Many people, however, feel it's not the right time for the following reasons:

Fear of addiction is why many doctors limit use of pharmacological drugs for terminal patients. That terminal patients might become substance abusers is absurd and insulting. To believe that the terminal patient would not like to leave this earth as a drug user demonstrates complete misunderstanding of the mechanism involved in substance abuse. Much of this misunderstanding has a cultural basis; drug abuse is a major social problem, and the use of narcotics has taken on negative connotations. The general public, too, has a bias against these drugs. Very few people know, however, that these drugs (morphine or similar drugs) are always used by doctors for the temporary relief of acute pain associated with any medical condition, to be discontinued when the patient has recovered from the acute condition. This is the case for severe chest pain associated with a heart attack, the discomfort following major surgery, a woman in labor, or even a severe cough. Many of these patients would be surprised if they knew that benign names such as Demerol, Codeine, or Dilaudid are really morphine or morphine-like substances.

The common belief is that repeated use of a narcotic by any person will automatically lead to addiction and permanent dependency on the drug. This is completely wrong. A drug addict is an emotionally disturbed person who expresses his disturbance through in drug addiction. If his emotional problems were not expressed through drug addition, they would be expressed in some other form such as criminal behavior, alcoholism, etc. A normal human being who, for some medical reason, is exposed to the extensive use of narcotics and then no longer needs them will have no trouble being weaned simply by decreasing the dosage progressively. Conversely, detoxification almost never works in a drug addict. Assuming the patient becomes addicted, and I do not deny that this can occasionally occur, this addiction is irrelevant given a patient's terminal condition. The horror of addiction is what happens to an addict over the long-term, and there is no long-term for dying patients.

Besides addiction, ignorance is another common reason why drugs aren't given to dying patients. Relatively few doctors, pharmacists, and pharmacologists understand how drugs affect dying patients. The general public has only a vague and negative idea of their real effect. Most people are unaware that a whole pharmacology of powerful drugs is available but not used to their full potential. Drugs often aren't administered properly at night or weekends in hospitals because fewer qualified personnel are on duty at these times. Because the exact nature of the diagnosis and prognosis is almost never discussed with the patient, the exact nature of the medication (morphine or morphine derivatives) is almost never discussed with the patient either. When the patient is informed that he is receiving narcotics, he is usually embarrassed.

Complicated regulations concerning the administration of large quantities of drugs also discourages their use. The fear is that these drugs could be sidetracked and used by addicts. Heroin, widely prescribed in other countries for terminal patients, is not legal in this country.

The attitudes and actions of caregivers, family and friends also prevent drugs from being administered effectively. They reason that dying patients always have had pain and anxiety, and perhaps pain and suffering when dying have some profound meaning. It may be that some people think that pain in dying is a kind of martyrdom that leads to a seat in Heaven. And there are patients who feel like cowards if they take drugs, believeing they're taking the easy way out rather than putting up a fight.

The most significant factor in our under-use of drugs, however, is the individual and societal fear of a repulsion for death. Our fear and anxiety is projected onto the dying person. The dying person deflects our fear—his pain and suffering draws all our attention and we don't have a chance for self-examination. If he were calm and accepting, it might cause us to confront our fear and wonder if we could die in a similar way.

Finally, there are the medicolegal considerations. One has to understand that doctors go by the book. The Food and Drug Administration requires that the indications and dosage of each specific medication be clearly codified. This has been done for the living but there are very few guidelines for the use of pharmacologic drugs in dying patients, and there is no wide statistical study for the specific use of each drug for each specific complaint presented by a terminal patient. Among the different factors that paralyze the medical profession is the fear of shortening a life (even by a few days) by overdose and being accused of murder.

Chapter 16

MANAGEMENT OF PAIN IN TERMINAL PATIENTS

"One of the worst aspects of cancer pain is that it is a constant reminder of the disease and death." —Jeanne Stover, Cancer Pain Panel
Member 1991-1992

While there are a number of painful, fatal diseases, cancer is the
one that causes the most pain for the most people, so much of the discussion in this chapter will revolve around this particular disease. Cancer kills one person in five in the United States and one person in ten
in the world. Out of a population of 240 million, the annual birth rate
and the death rate in the USA are about 1% (2.5 million births and 2.5
million deaths). One million cases of cancer are diagnosed in the United
States each year causing a half-million deaths. Physical pain and mental
depression are often associated with advanced cancer. About 75% of patients with advanced cancer have pain, and this pain certainly impairs
the quality of life of a cancer patient.

The individual perception of pain and appreciation of its meaning are complex phenomena that involve psychological processes in addition to activation of nociceptive pathways. These phenomena would
explain placebo analgesia and even acupuncture. Pain intensity is not
proportional to the type or extent of tissue damage.

It's astonishing that elderly patients, especially, are undertreated
given that we possess the drugs and treatment experience necessary to
relieve most if not all of their pain. Because we don't and their pain is
often uncontrolled, they often feel helpless and suicidal (and sometimes
actually attempt suicide). Clinicians should reassure patients and family that pain can be controlled safely and effectively, and that it is their
responsibility to ask that the pain be controlled.

It is important to individualize treatment and to start with the sim-
plest and least invasive mode. Commonly available drugs with dosage
and directions for use are listed at the end of this chapter. This list fol-

lows the World Health Organization (WHO) guidelines.

Placebos

Hippocrates noted that some patients are cured solely through a good rapport with the physician; this, I suppose was the first placebo. The history of medicine is, in effect, a history of placebos since it is only in recent years that real drugs have been introduced. Much of the treatment in the past was innocuous or dangerous with the exception of opium for pain, digitalis for heart failure, cinchona bark for malaria and lime juice for scurvy.

Despite their limited power in the past, physicians always have been respected for their ability to cure. The placebo response is common and its analgesic effect may be mediated to a great extent through endogenous opioid pathways. Placebos, if effective, are effective only for a short time and should not be used for extensive management of cancer pain.

Medication to a dying patient is a blessing but it is not a substitute for a concerned doctor. Both are necessary. Tremendous emotional pain occurs because patients fear doctors are abandoning them or because this abandonment actually takes place. Very few doctors spend enough time listening or talking to terminal patients. Rather than establish a meaningful relationship, they find some excuse to cut conversations short. Typically, doctors hand off terminal patients to specialists. They also prescribe tranquilizers for the surrounding family. This isn't necessarily a bad idea, but it can also lead to avoiding facing the emotional realities of the situation.

The Goals of Cancer Pain Management

Improving cancer treatment with surgery, chemotherapy and/or radiotherapy has extended patients' lives but also created numerous complications. People are more aware of the disease's progressive nature—the improved treatment process gives people more time to reflect on the nature of the disease and the inevitability of death—and thus become more fearful. On top of that, the new treatments create socioeconomic problems that exacerbate patients' anxieties.

Dying in pain and grief is a neglected topic although it is the most dramatic stress encountered by individuals in their lifetime. If pain and suffering are intolerable and incapacitating, they should be treated like any other disease mostly by pharmacological drugs and/or any other support by the family and caregivers.

Death with dignity can be achieved only by relieving pain and anxiety. Amazingly, this simple fact is not widely understood or accepted. The combination of pharmacological drugs and support from family and caregivers is the answer. Unfortunately, not enough people are asking the right questions. The relative few who have (Kübler-Ross, 1969, 1975) have helped us begin to view death as a separate entity. We must start dealing with a dying patient as a candidate for death in the same way we deal with a pregnant woman as a candidate for birth. This may call for medical (pharmacologic) treatment or another type of treatment for which the average physician (or even specialist) is not always qualified. This is because medical and surgical oncologists are in the forefront of medical management to cure cancer or extend life <u>and nothing else</u>. Yet they find themselves asked to respond to the pain and anxiety of the dying patient as well as of the family—a response for which they haven't been trained.

Treatment of cancer pain always has been limited, and the most frequent medications for pain on a chemotherapy ward were, and sometimes still are only Tylenol for pain and Dalmane for sleeping. The pain of a malignant disease is usually not very severe at least not in the early stage, but it is the chronic, prolonged duration of the disease that makes it difficult to manage. Depression and anxiety magnify the pain associated with this type of disease.

Many patients dying of cancer do so only after weeks and months of uncontrolled pain. Many hospitalized patients die in pain and even in severe pain. The main reason for poor pain control is undertreatment. Many patients and doctors believe nothing can be done to relieve this pain for reasons that are misguided at best and completely wrong at worst.

Reviews of the literature shows that addiction, rapid escalation of dosage and impairment of mental faculties do not exist when cancer pain is adequately treated. A lack of in-depth clinical research with comparative series about the relief of pain and anxiety in cancer patients, however, prevents hospitals and doctors from changing their pain management policies. This is because the problem of terminally ill patients in pain presents a dilemma. On the one hand, we wish to provide adequate analgesia. On the other hand, we do not wish to hasten death by causing a depression of vital functions. Further, we also would like an active and alert patient without depression, anxiety, or distress. The solution to this dilemma is relatively simple: Assemble a pain control team composed of a surgeon, neurosurgeon, anesthesiologist, and psychiatrist. This team has the right mix of experience and expertise to relieve pain and anxiety without harming vital functions.

In advanced cases, especially with anxiety and depression, it may take this team three to four weeks for satisfactory pain control, though two to four days should be the norm. The team should have three successive goals:

1. A pain-free patient and a restful night.
2. Freedom from pain with movement in bed.
3. Freedom of pain with movement out of bed.

When pain expands and dominates one's existence, life isn't worth living. Contrary to acute pain, chronic cancer pain has no end and it becomes worse rather than better. Because cancer pain is continuous, the treatment should be continuous—preventative rather than based on the patient's request.

A learning curve must be climbed before the medical profession can confidently assure patients that severe pain in advanced cancer can be controlled. The pharmacology of pain for advanced cancer has nothing to do with the pharmacology of acute pain for non-cancer patients. Cancer pain is not relieved by mild analgesics. A short life expectancy necessitates prescribing strong narcotics. Most patients with terminal cancer have more than one symptom, and adjuvant therapy is necessary.

Diversionary activity such as backrubs, craft work, books, radio and television, dayroom activities and someone to talk to is important. Pain is worse when it occupies the patient's whole attention, and so these non-medical aspects of treatment should be incorporated into the overall plan.

THE TECHNOLOGY OF DRUG DELIVERY

We now have the ability to provide patients with self-administered pain medication through continuous intravenous (IV) lines; they no longer need to rely on others or to suffer and wait until caregivers recognize that they need more medication. Experience with this type of continuous sedation has been studied mostly with postoperative patients, but the results can be easily extended to terminal patients in pain. The great advantage is that there is continuous action and therefore no significant fluctuations in drug level. Consequently, there's more efficient sedation and less habituation to drugs. With more research and experience, we can make this on-demand medication an even more effective tool to ease the pain and suffering of terminal patients. In fact, there's absolutely no reason why we would confine its use to the final weeks of these patients' lives; it can be instituted much earlier. We already possess and are using the technology of permanent intravenous lines with constant infusion pumps. Patients with intractable pain can be discharged with such a device.

DRUGS FOR THE MANAGEMENT OF PAIN IN CANCER PATIENTS

Here is a concise list of the various medications for the management of cancer patients. Patients and concerned families should be made aware of what is available. It may surprise you to learn that not all physicians treating terminal patients know this list. I am not saying that patients or families should take over the physician's role, but an alert and sophisticated patient helps physicians do their jobs well.

EARLY STAGES OF PAIN

One can always start with sodium salicylate (aspirin) or acetaminophen (Excedrin). Salicylates are gastric irritants and may lead to gastric ulcers. They can also interfere with the coagulation of blood. Diflunisal (Dolobid) is a salicylic acid derivative but is less of a gastric irritant. Magnesium salicylate (Magan, Mobidin), choline magnesium trisalicylate (Trilisate), and salsalate (salicylosalicylic acid or Mono-Gesic) may have fewer side-effects on blood coagulation. Serious complications are frequent (mostly perforated ulcer) possibly because of the widespread use of these medications. Sucralfate and misoprostol (antiulcer medications) are used to prevent and treat the gastric irritation produced by the salicylates. Coating (cimetidine) is not very effective.

Frequent use of aspirin can also lead to bone marrow depression and bleeding. Allergy to aspirin is also frequent.

Acetaminophen has effects similar to aspirin, with few side-effects (no gastric irritation and no allergy). Gastric absorption, however, is slower.

MILD-TO-MODERATE PAIN

The choices are numerous and the list is increasing. Frequent change of medication and numerous trials and errors will finally lead to the proper selection. Usually the following NSAIDs (nonsteroid antiinflammatory drugs) become necessary:

1. The most common NSAIDs are Rimadyl, Arthropan, Lodine, Nalfon, Orudis, Toradol (oral or intramuscular), Meclomen, Ponstel, Anaprox, and Ibuprofen. Motrin is the only non-prescription NSAID.

2. The acetic acid derivations are powerful but may be toxic. Indomethacin (Indocin) is anti-inflammatory and analgesic. Sulindac (clinoril) has long-term effect and is less toxic. Tolmetin is similar to aspirin but less toxic. Ketorolac (Toradol) is a powerful analgesic. New class of NSAIDs are phenylacetic acid derivatives (diclofenac, fenclofenac, alclofenac) which can be combined with aspirin.

3. The propionic acid derivatives are Naproxen (Naprosyn, Anaprox) which are less toxic than aspirin and indomethacin. The profens such as Fenoprofen (Naflon), Flurbiprofen (Ansaid), Ibuprofen (Nuprin), Etoprofen (Orudis) are more tolerated and more active and can be com-

bined with other NSAIDs.

4. Oxicam derivatives are represented by Piroxicam (Feldene). It is long acting.

5. Pyrazoles derivatives are represented by Phenylbutazone, a good analgesic, but it has bone marrow toxicity.

NSAIDS are a heterogenous group of drugs, not always chemically related. They are best known for their relief of pain in inflammation and arthritic conditions; their analgesic role in other types of pain continues to grow. Contrary to opiates (see later) which are for acute pain, NSAIDs are for chronic pain and for pain due to a malignant origin. These are easily combined with other sedatives.

NSAIDS are generally prescribed for chronic pain because of low abuse potential and their very limited tolerance when compared to opiates (Day, et al., 1987). The pharmacology of these drugs has been studied mostly in osteoarthritis of the elderly. These medications are effective when given in the right dose, through the right route and at the proper time.

The complications and contraindications of NSAIDs are renal failure, hepatic dysfunction, bleeding and gastric ulceration.

All these drugs have similar efficacy. Only experience will guide the clinician in the selection. Each physician has his own preferred drugs. The prescribing physician should not hesitate to combine these drugs.

MODERATE-TO-SEVERE PAIN

When pain persists or increases, add to NSAIDS (do not substitute) a mild opioid such as codeine (methylmorphine) or a codeine derivative such as hydrocodone (Hycodan) or oxycodone (Percodan). Preparation can combine NSAIDs and opioids but watch for NSAIDs toxicity, especially in the elderly. Aspirin or acetaminophen can also be combined with codeine derivatives such as hydrocodone (Lorcet, Lortab, Vicodin, etc.) or oxycodone (Roxicodone, Percocet, Tylox, etc.). The purpose of adding codeine and the like is not to exceed the maximum dose of toxicity in NSAIDs and acetaminophen.

Persistent Moderate-to-Severe Pain (or severe pain from onset)

The treatment is to increase the dosage of opioids to potency. They are the most frequently used for cancer pain because they are effective, easy to titrate, and have a favorable risk-to-benefit ratio.

a. Classification of Opioids. There is no ceiling to their analgesic efficacy and they will not reverse or antagonize the effects of other opioids. The usual opioids are:

Morphine. It is not used for chronic conditions except for widespread malignancies. For pain due to widespread cancer, oral administration every four hours is recommended. The daily dose for patients with widespread cancer varies from 60 to 1800mg with an average of 240mg/day. The routes are oral, rectal suppositories or subcutaneously.

Meperidine (Pethidine or Demerol) is less potent than morphine and larger doses are needed. Given continuously by intramuscular or intravenous route is as effective as oral therapy for prolonged treatment. Elderly patients appear to be more sensitive to Demerol. It is contraindicated for prolonged treatment.

Fentanyl can be used as a transdermal preparation.

Methadone is a synthetic substitute of morphine. It is long acting and can be taken orally.

Hydromorphone (Dilaudid) can be used rectally.

Diamorphine (heroin) is not used in the United States.

Codeine (or methylmorphine) and derivatives, as previously noted, are relatively mild opiates.

Agonist-antagonists: Pentazocine, Buprenorphine, Butorphanol, and Nalbuphine are like morphine but less addictive.

b. Tolerance. Tolerance and physical dependence on opioids are expected with long-term use and should not be confused with psychological dependency (addiction) manifested in drug abuse behavior. This confusion contributes to ineffective treatment and to the problem of undertreatment. Rarely do cancer patients exhibit the drug abuse behavior of addiction. When opioid administration has to be discontinued (in case of a good response to chemotherapy and/or radiotherapy), progressive withdrawal within a week presents no problem.

Tolerance is defined as the need to increase dose requirement over time to maintain pain relief. The first sign is a decrease in the duration of analgesia for a given dose. Increasing dose requirements are usually correlated with progressive disease which produces increased pain intensity. Patients with stable disease do not usually require increasing dose.

c. Dosage. To allow pain to reemerge before administering the next dose not only produces anxiety but increases suffering and leads to drug tolerance. Therefore, medication should be administered regularly in a *preventive* manner. The next dose should be given before the previous one has worn off. This is the only way to *erase the memory and fear of pain*. The correct dose is the one that gives relief. Maximums are not applicable in advanced cancer. Dosage is individualized to achieve pain relief with limited adverse effect. There is practically no ceiling for opioid agonist: several hundred milligrams of morphine every 4 hours may be needed for severe pain. Before switching routes of administration it is better to use different drugs sequentially. For instance, switch from morphine to Dilaudid, etc.

d. Routes of administration. In general, the oral route is preferred but, if contraindicated, use the rectal or transdermal route. The oral route is preferred although the dosage is higher than when other routes are used in view of intestinal and liver metabolism and although it is slow acting. The oral route requires therefore specific titration. It is the most convenient and cost effective. For the oral route, tablets, capsules, or liquid are available in immediate or control-released forms. When the patient is unable to swallow or to take medication orally (in case of oral mucositis mostly during the last month of life), the doctor can try rectal or transdermal route.

Rectal route is used when nausea or vomiting is present: morphine, hydromorphine (Dilaudid), and oxymorphine (Numorphan) are available as suppositories.

Transdermal route, Fentanyl (Duragesic transdermal); and nasal route, butorphanol (Stadol nasal spray) are also available.

Intravenous (IV) or subcutaneous (SC) routes may produce local irritation. Continuous infusion is used mostly when high dose is needed, that is, in preterminal or terminal patients. It is the most rapid.

The intramuscular route is to be avoided as much as possible because it is painful, inconvenient and unreliable.

e. Management of side-effects. There are great individual variations. One has to watch for the side-effects of drugs because they may panic the patient and the surrounding family. Doctors have to be as careful and familiar with drugs in terminal patients as in any other patients.

Constipation is common and is to be differentiated from intestinal obstruction or paralytic ileus. For mild constipation, increased fiber or a mild laxative, such as Milk of Magnesia, should be taken regularly. For severe constipation due to inhibition of intestinal peristalsis by opioids, a cathartic such as bisacodyl or senna concentrate or hyperosmotic agents (lactulose or sorbitol) is needed. These medications should be taken orally at bedtime or by suppository in early morning. Stool softeners or emollient laxatives have limited indications.

Sedation with a tendency to sleep is temporary and can be seen with high dosage of opioids. Alertness can be increased with caffeine, dextro-amphetamine (Dexedrine), pemoline, or methylphenidate (Ritalin) which improves memory and concentration.

Nausea and vomiting are controlled with antiemetics, such as metoclopramide, prochlorperazine, chlorpromazine or haloperidol. Respiratory depression needs the use of opioid antagonist such as titrated Naloxone given intravenously with glucose in water. Watch for sudden reversal of the sedation effect of opioids.

Other side-effects, such as seizures and myoclonus, hallucination, confusion, sexual dysfunction (common male complaint), sleep disturbance, and pruritus, require specific treatment and careful dosage.

Urinary retention is to be carefully monitored.

Fear of killing the patient by respiratory depression or cardiac arrest is usually unfounded because of tolerance, but the clinician is frequently concerned, and this is the reason for undertreatment. The administration of any medication is always a risk-versus-benefit consideration. When the patient's death is imminent due to the progression of the primary disease, an increased risk of earlier death *counts little* against the benefit of pain relief and painless death. The ethical duty of relieving pain by increasing the dose of medication should be *more important* than the fear of shortening life by a few days. The person dying of cancer should not be obligated to live out life with unrelieved pain because of the doctor's fear of side-effects, and appropriate aggressive palliation should be given.

St. Christopher's and St. Joseph's Hospice in London

The British started the hospice concept of total care of the terminally ill patient including medical, social, psychological, and spiritual (religious) care. In the hospice, the British have a more enlightened approach to the use of drugs, especially for people dying of cancer. Although only half of all cancer patients experience pain of any significance, intractable pain is the most common reason for hospitalization of cancer patients.

The British mostly use diacetyl morphine (diamorphine or heroin). Diamorphine mixed with cocaine is given by mouth every four hours, combined with chlorpromazine (anti-nausea and to reinforce pain relief). It is given parenterally (IV or SC) if there is difficulty in swallowing. The relief of pain is usually immediate, but sometimes it takes up to 2 weeks. Diamorphine is preferable to morphine because it does not produce nausea-vomiting, does not affect appetite, enhances the mood of the patients (they become almost *euphoric*), stops coughs, and relieves anxiety. The dose is 5 to 100 mg (usually 30) every four hours. There has been no double blind study, however. The disadvantage is that it is highly addictive with rapid tolerance. However, if an adequate dose is given on a regular schedule, there is no addiction.

If necessary, the narcotic (diamorphine or heroin) should be combined with antidepressants, anxiolytics, and steroids. Very few patients die of cancer with pain at St. Christopher's and St. Joseph's Hospice.

Other Modes of Therapy

"Cancer Pain Can Be Relieved (1988)," a booklet for patients and family, is available on request from the Wisconsin Cancer Pain Initiative, and lists other modes of therapy.

1. Adjuvant drugs:

· Corticosteroids (Dexamethasone) are anti-inflammatory, anti-emetic, stimulate appetite, and elevate mood. They are beneficial in cachexia and anorexia of terminal patients. They reduce intracranial pressure and edema.

· Anticonvulsants are used in neuropathic pain, especially when associated with lancing and burning. Usual drugs are Phenytoin, carbamazepine, valproate, and clonazepam.

2. Acupuncture, accupressure, cutaneous stimulation, and superficial heat can be used.

3. Psychotherapy, peer support group, and pastoral counseling are of benefit when requested.

4. Hypnosis, yoga, biofeedback, and use of ice can modify or abolish the experience of pain and are always beneficial for those who believe in them.

TREATMENT OF INTRACTABLE PAIN

Once in a while, a cancer pain may become resistant to any and all medications. In this case, various kinds of semi-invasive or invasive surgical procedures becomes necessary. These procedures should be used more often:

1. Invasive Surgery for Palliation

· Radiotherapy for bone metastases

· Nerve blocks

· Catheter placement for continuous drug delivery

- Neurosurgery (neuroablation):
- peripheral neurectomy
- dorsal rhizotomy
- anterolateral cordotomy
- commissural myelotomy

2. Regional Anesthesia

Neurolytic agents are less popular today: the common agents are alcohol, phenol and hypertonic saline. The neurolysis can be done on the spinal cord, on the celiac plexus, or around the nerves.

Electrical deep brain stimulation is very often helpful in severe cases.

Intrathecal, spinal, or epidural morphine can be effective.

Subarachnoid or epidural implantation of catheter can continuously deliver the sedative in the spinal fluid. These catheter implantations usually last days or weeks, but with a modern apparatus, they can last for years.

Long-acting narcotics such as methadone and morphine administration in a continuous IV infusion ensure adequate analgesia for terminal patients in the hospital or even at home.

Chapter 17

DIAGNOSIS AND TREATMENT OF DEPRESSION
IN DYING PATIENTS

Quos vult perdere Jupiter dementat—When Gods want to destroy people, they render them insane. —Latin Quotation

Indeed, it sometimes seems that dying people are in a state of near insanity. At least this is how they appear to those surrounding them. Typically, family and friends keep a distance from them, as if death is some contagious disease that the living have to protect themselves from. This strange state of mind creates an abyss between the living and the dying. They don't talk to each other in meaningful ways, and this makes it difficult to change perceptions. It also makes it difficult for terminal patients to escape their depression.

Terminal patients, unlike most other people, don't ask for help to relieve their depression. Other patients are willing to discuss with their doctor the nature and cause of their depression. Terminally ill people, on the other hand, are reluctant or unwilling to address their coming death as the cause of their depression. Even if these people are willing to talk about it, they rarely find a receptive ear. Everyone is busy fighting rather than coming to terms with death. Because the terminal patient is isolated and unable to discuss the coming death with anyone, death and the feelings it engenders (fear, depression, anxiety) are ignored and remain untreated. This is true even though we have drugs that can treat these emotional ills with relative ease.

In fact, the problem is not so much what medication to use, but rather to listen when terminal patients talk about their depression and have the courage and the determination to treat them aggressively. Consciously or not, many doctors don't recognize how serious this depression and how necessary it is to treat it. We can provide relief for depression and anxiety in terminal patients and their families, but we're going to have to overcome a bias against such treatment and a willingness to learn more about what's most effective.

We need to begin learning about the best ways to treat depression and anxiety in terminal patients rather than simply prescribing the same drugs we would for others. The worst thing that could happen is for a practicing physician to treat people who are dying with powerful drugs without the proper knowledge and experience.

Statistics show that the severe mental symptoms presented by dying patients are ignored or at least undertreated, and these patients are denied treatment that is easily available and badly needed. One in eight individuals requires treatment for depression during their active life, and most of these patients receive the proper treatment. But seven out of eight dying patients are depressed during their last weeks or months of life, and most of them don't receive treatment for it.

Part of the problem is that we falsely assume that psychiatrists should manage terminal symptomatology (fear, anxiety, depression) and not the patient's treating physician. While the symptoms may be in the psychiatrist's area of expertise, the treatment of people who are dying is outside of it (The only possible exception would be a psychiatrist highly specialized in psychopharmacology). The general care physician usually has much more experience with dying patients as well as greater familiarity with the patient (and thus can read his or her mood better). A combination of psychotherapy and medication usually works well, especially if the depression and anxiety is recognized early and treated aggressively. Unfortunately, most of the time it is recognized late in the process and treated tentatively.

Depression occurs in almost 10% of elderly patients in the general population over 65 years of age, even when not terminally ill. Terminal conditions make depression worse. Almost 80% of elderly terminal patients are depressed. Psychological symptoms of depression in the elderly may be difficult to distinguish from senile dementia, Alzheimer's disease and other organic diseases. Disorientation, loss of memory and irritability are also worse in terminal patients. In view of poor blood circulation in the elderly, the effective dosage of medication often needs to be lowered. Many medications, such as cardiovascular drugs, hormone drugs, psychotropic drugs, anti-cancer drugs and anti-inflammatory antibiotics can cause depression or have associated symptoms as a side-effect.

Prevailing social norms not only causes terminal patients to be reluctant to talk about their depression, but it causes caregivers to be reluctant to initiate and maintain treatment; it also causes them to discontinue treatment if it seems there is a little improvement. Discrimination against terminal patients may not be conscious, but there is definitely de facto discrimination. We need to talk more about these issues so that doctors, nurses and the public are educated about the emotional trauma dying patients go through and what's needed to relieve their emotional pain.

How and Why Dying People Feel The Way They Do

Depression is an abnormal reaction to a difficult situation. It can start with sadness, which is a normal reaction to a contrary experience if it doesn't last long. It becomes real depression when apathy, anxiety, profound sadness and loss of pleasure and enjoyment of life (anhedonia) are added and these feelings persist.

What's significant is that depression and talk of suicide are the second most common reason for terminal patients to be hospitalized (the most common reason is to prolong life). Depression and associated symptoms among those who are dying are so common, in fact, that they have become the definition of a terminal condition. If a terminal patient is not depressed, fearful or anxious, the surrounding people (including the medical profession) consider it abnormal.

Psychotic traits, hallucinations and delusions may also appear in depressed patients who are dying. Melancholy, loss of energy or agitation, oversleeping or insomnia and phobias are also common. Panic attacks and anxiety disorders are other emotional ills frequently associated with depression. Social phobia (fear of isolation or real isolation) is typical. Anorexia nervosa is more frequent than bulimia and may play a role in weight loss. The picture may be complicated with irritability, poor concentration, indecisiveness, loss of sexual interest, self pity and pessimism. Conversion hysteria or somatization disorder is a frequent cause of misdiagnosis.

Many of these symptoms are nothing more than the consequences of depression and anxiety. Each one should be addressed specifically: melancholia, guilt, panic, mania, sadness, fear and mood disorders. It's been said that dying patients are in a state of near-insanity, but what hasn't been said is that this is a result of untreated depression. It's neither natural nor inevitable that terminal patients experience these awful symptoms. Too often, however, they're isolated by their loved ones and are reluctant to seek or continue treatment for their depression.

Suicide in Advanced Cancer

The problem of euthanasia will be approached in a subsequent chapter. Dying patients who commit suicide or request euthanasia do so simply because they're in severe physical pain or because of depression. Relatively few terminal cancer patients commit suicide if the above two problems are solved, and it's a mistake to believe that this is a common reaction. Still, we need to treat suicidal, terminal patients in more effective ways. Perhaps the most effective treatment is to attack the physical pain and depression simultaneously. We know from studies that when this is done, requests for euthanasia decrease.

Most persons (oral type, passive-dependent personality) who use medication as a mode of suicide are frightened of pain and violence. They want a simple and quick exit, like sleep, and the pill offers the kind of painless death they wish.

There are terminal patients, however, who want to end their life, even when physical pain or depression don't exist. They just lose interest, and since they're going to die soon it may as well be now rather than later. Many are aware of the impositions they make on others and want to remove that burden. Most of them are withdrawn and do not get involved in deep discussion on this subject.

You can't treat a terminal patient's depression the way you would another person with this emotional illness. People who are dying and depressed deserve special treatment, and we need to recognize that their terminal condition warrants it. Let's start with the double-edged sword of treating depressed, dying patients. On the one hand, doctors are inclined to take more risks and be more aggressive in treating these patients knowing that they'll soon die no matter what they do. On the other hand, they refrain from doing anything, fearing that anything they do might kill the patient; doctors are terrified of prescribing a treatment in which a complication or side-effect could shorten the patient's life.

This is true not only in the treatment of depression but in any type of treatment for these patients. During my career I have seen acutely ill patients who died in the middle of vigorous medical or surgical procedures and their death was classified as a calculated risk of the procedures. If a terminal patient dies in the middle of a similar vigorous treatment, ethical and even legal issues are raised. The fear of terminating an already terminal life is widespread, and it often clouds the judgment of caregivers.

This fear should not interfere with case management, otherwise proper treatment can be difficult or even impossible. The terminal patient will die whether or not he is taking medication. One has to be practical. The best course of action is to inform the patient and/or family in lay terms about the rare but possible eventuality of death with the administration of a strong drug. A recent Supreme Court ruling allows doctors to take such a risk. The worst thing to do is give up on dying patients with the excuse that one is concerned about the side-effects of the medication.

The concern about how dying people would react to specific medication can also hamper treatment. The question "How is he going to react to the medication?" really means, "How am I going to react if he behaves in a way I cannot deal with, if he loses control, which in turn will make me lose control?" It's not that doctors aren't concerned about the depression of dying patients; it's that their concern is opposed by stronger forces. Doctors are not immune to the following psychological process: We spend our lives ignoring and refusing to think about death, and we become fearful that a dying person will oblige us to think about facing death. Thus, we try to convince them that they are in good health, we behave as if they are not dying or we run away from them. We expect dying patients to be brave in the face of death and to fight it to the bitter end. We forget that most of the time these expectations are unrealistic, and we selfishly demand that a terminal patient handle the emotional turmoil produced around him. He can't, and depression and anxiety are often the result.

We lack a systematic approach to the various emotional problems presented by terminal patients. A treatment regimen with medication has not been systematized, analyzed, coordinated and regulated. Consequently, the physician responsible for dealing with a terminal patient has to make up his own mind about treatment. Without a systematic process, doctors often procrastinate when faced with this issue.

In treating depression and associated symptoms of terminal patients, the goals are completely different from those of non-terminal patients. For instance, one should not be concerned about:

- Tolerance of medication.
- Hypothetical addiction.
- Stigma attached to depression (and mental illness in general) and its management.
- Detoxification and eventual discontinuance of medication.
- Maintenance therapy.
- Family interference.
- The long-term effects or complications of treatment.

The goal is restoration of psychological and psychosocial functions, coming to terms with one's condition, achieving a calm, peaceful mood and being able to make rational decisions about important matters (wills, funerals, etc.).

Because of a lack of testing, doctors don't have good guidelines about the best drugs to use with depressed, terminal patients. We do know, however, that certain drugs are effective in treating depression generally, and we should start with them as well as proven therapeutic strategies. Commonly available drugs with dosage and directions for use are listed at the end of this chapter.

The P.R.N. Medication Orders

A p.r.n. medication order means "as needed." The treating physician specifies the dose of the medication and the frequency of administration, but leaves it to the nurse to make a determination and to the patient to request the medication if needed. Almost all sedatives or sleeping medications are p.r.n. orders. If the patient does not complain of pain or is sleeping, the medication is not administered. The purpose of the p.r.n. order is to cut the amount of medication by administering it only when really needed. Unfortunately, this order often results in neglect. The administration of p.r.n. orders depends on how busy the hospital staff is, how many nurses cover the floor, the moods of the nurses and how determined the patient is.

Because of these variables, p.r.n. orders are often neglected, especially at night and on weekends and especially if patients are dying. Terminal patients are withdrawn, insecure and sometimes ignored by doctors and nurses who are too busy saving lives. Terminal patients are usually not a high-priority; their placement in rooms at the end of the hall epitomizes how the hospital staff views them. They're also undertreated because any treatment might be the final straw.

All of this contributes to the depression and anxiety of hospitalized people who don't have long to live. They feel isolated and ignored, and they often don't receive the medication they should receive—medication that might improve how they feel physically and emotionally.

Psychotherapy of Terminal Patients

Medication alone is not enough; feelings of guilt, worthlessness, helplessness, and hopelessness also need to be treated through psychotherapy. Very few therapists have much experience in treating dying patients. The experience of psychiatrists dealing with terminal patients is so limited that whenever one of them deals in depth with one or two such patients he either reports it in a psychiatric journal or even writes a book about it. Typically, social workers rather than psychologists or psychiatrists counsel the dying patient and family, but even this counseling is often done seat-of-the-pants style. Most psychotherapy focuses on symptom amelioration—dealing with depression and all its different clinical features. It is usually time-limited and not always effective, especially in the elderly and terminal patients. It works more effectively when combined with medication. In fact, psychotherapy and drugs reinforce each other and some form of psychotherapy, or at least counseling (just listening), should always accompany drug prescription.

We also need to dovetail treatment to the needs of individual patients. Some terminal patients with mild to moderate depression may only need psychotherapy; some patients may also have objection to drugs to treat their depression. From a practical point of view, the mental health practitioner should engage in supportive therapy to provide advice and guidance on current problems, reinforcement of psychological strength and development of social support.

Psychoanalysis of the dying is virgin territory. Nobody really knows what goes on in their minds. We assume that what they're thinking about, we'd be thinking about if we were dying. This assumption, however, is based only on observation; we rarely explore and analyze in any depth what dying people are feeling, and they have no incentive to be forthcoming. Historically, few psychoanalysts (or anyone else, for that matter) have devoted significant time or effort to this subject; even Freud and Jung treat this issue somewhat superficially. It's also true that many years ago, the dying process took relatively little time, providing scant opportunity for in-depth analysis. In addition, there were larger social problems that took precedence; investigating what went on in the minds of the dying would have seemed like a trivial endeavor.

Today, we avoid this subject because we believe that terminal patients are scared of expressing their true feelings. In fact, we're the ones who are frightened of moving into this taboo territory. Even therapists are fearful of this subject (they're human too), though they might be willing to work with a dying patient if that patient's doctor, family or the patient himself requested this intervention. This never happens.

While hearing the innermost thoughts and feelings of a dying person might strike some as morbid, it also holds tremendous interest for us all. Who doesn't want to ask a million questions such as:

· What does it feel like to be leaving all your loved ones, your friends and the world behind?

· Are you scared; what frightens you the most; do you feel at peace or a sense of acceptance and calm?

· Do you worry about the afterlife? If there is one, where would you be after you die?

· What do you dream about?

· Looking back, is there anything you wish you had done differently; what are you most proud of?

It takes courage to ask these questions and listen to the answers, and the only one who I know has done so is Mitch Albom in his book, *Tuesdays with Morrie* (Doubleday, 1997). The author's former teacher is dying of amyotrophic lateral sclerosis (ALS), and he talks with Morrie about every subject under the sun as his life ebbs. It's a very moving story as Morrie conveys his life through the perspective of approaching death. While Morrie certainly is courageous in talking about his life, the author is even more courageous in one sense, in that he has the fortitude and interest to listen.

If we all could listen and receive valuable insights from the dying, we would be that much more prepared to accept our own deaths. I have met a few Morries in my career, and I related some of their stories in an earlier chapter. I listened with what Kirkegaard described as fear and trembling as they talked to me about how they were feeling, not just physically but emotionally. Sometimes it was difficult to listen, and there were times when I lacked the courage (as well as the time) to sit while a dying person unburdened himself. I've watched other health-care professionals do the same thing.

The problem isn't that we need more Morries in the world willing to talk; it's that we need more Mitches to listen and record what the Morries say. The challenge, perhaps, is for both the living and the dying.

Both need to open up to each other.

Two to three weeks after a loved one's death, profound bereavement, suicidal thoughts, and profound guilt are common among family members (Goldberg et al., 1986). One fourth of widows show signs of major depression two months after the death of a loved one and require medication. Besides depression, there is suicidal ideation, poor health and inability to keep a job. Associated symptoms are lethargy, insomnia, loss of appetite, fatigue and somatic complaints such as headaches, dizziness and blurred vision. Many more bereaved people than commonly thought are taking medication for grief. Today, almost two-thirds of all widows use anti-depressants.

Acute grief is characterized by recurrent episodes of anxiety during which the dead person is strongly missed and this anxiety usually lasts for two weeks. Barbiturates and tranquilizers are the classic drugs administered, but Kübler-Ross (1973) suggests a screaming room where the bereaved can cry and scream in the presence of an understanding nurse or religious minister. All too often it is the doctor's intolerance of this loud anguish that leads to the prescription of sedatives. St. Christopher's Hospice in London has a post-bereavement family service support, though most churches and ministers aren't involved in this post-bereavement process as they were in the past.

Healthcare providers have a significant impact on the grief of mourners and how difficult the bereavement period is for them. If they provide a high standard of care for terminal patients, they give loved ones the precious memory of a dignified, peaceful death. This helps relieve the guilt of the bereaved: relief of physical pain and anxiety make death easier for the dying as well as for loved ones because everyone can empathize with the dying patient; everyone knows he or she is going to die one day. If the family is involved in the terminal care, this too helps relieve some of the guilt.

No systematic study has been made of the pharmacotherapy of the bereaved. It is possible that psychopharmacologic treatment of the bereaved is harmful, at least according to Freud (1917). Deutsch (1937) states this treatment only delays bereavement and most likely in a harmful way. Many other authors (Lindemann 1944; Maddison and Raphael 1973; Parkes 1964; Paul and Grosser 1965; Volkan and Showalter 1968) speak of a delayed reaction in the bereaved. Kübler-Ross (1973) suggests caution in drug use and only as an adjuvant and not a substitute for human care. Finally, there is always fear of addiction.

It is difficult to determine if grief is a normal process or an illness. It is accepted today that part of the grief is guilt, self-blame, anger toward the doctors and the dying person. Early grief (normal) shows three symptoms: depression or anxiety, sleeplessness, and crying. These symptoms usually diminish within four months. Suicidal thoughts, loss of interest and persistent guilt are not frequent. Anger, hostility and irritability often signal that someone is stuck in the grieving process.

It is accepted today that average grief should be treated with minor antidepressants such as benzodiazepine (diazepam, etc.). Major antidepressants are indicated only if grief is severe. Weaning should start within a month.

Sleeplessness is treated with hypnotic medications such as Flurazepam (Dalmane), temazepam (Restoril), triazolam (Halcion), which are all benzodiazepines. The risk is tolerance and habituation and the dose should be diminished after one week. Tricyclic antidepressants can also be helpful.

Again, what I find unacceptable is that, today, depressed people who are not mourning are freely treated with generous amounts of antidepressants (Prozac, for instance), sometimes for very long periods. When it comes to treating a depressed mourner similarly, hesitation arises on the part of the treating doctor as well as the people surrounding the mourner. It seems to me that there is a widespread masochistic concept that mourners should be depressed and to relieve their depression with drugs is almost betrayal of the deceased.

DRUGS FOR THE MANAGEMENT OF
DEPRESSION IN TERMINAL PATIENTS

HISTORY OF ANTIDEPRESSANTS:

From time immemorial humans have searched for ways to relieve physical pain, anxiety, and insomnia. The first effective therapy was and still is alcohol and opiates. In the 19th century, bromides were discovered. In the early 20th century, barbiturates were predominant. In the mid 20th century, tranquilizers (Meprobamate, Equanil, Miltown) became popular until it was realized that they were really not different from barbiturates. The most recent are the anxiolytics and hypnotics (benzodiazepines or BZD), the non-benzodiazepines - pure anxiolytics, and the non-benzodiazepines - pure hypnotics. The older drugs have side effects, but this is less serious when a person is dying. The modern anxiolytics are more efficient, have fewer side-effects, and pose less risk of overdose. There are still problems with tolerance, dependency, and withdrawal symptoms, although these are much less intense in terminal patients and not important anyway when a person is dying.

ANTIDEPRESSANT DRUGS

1) Tricyclics (TRAs) are amitriptyline, imipramine, desipramine, and nortriptyline (good start).

Amitriptyline, the oldest, is given intramuscularly, and Doxepin (like amitriptyline) is taken by mouth; they can produce hypotension. Imipramine (Tofranil) and Trimipramine are like Doxepin. Desipramine does not produce hypotension and can be taken in the morning. Nortriptyline is indicated for the elderly.

The first generation of tricyclics are the tertiary amine compounds (amitriptyline, imipramine) with many side-effects. Secondary amines (desipramine, nortriptyline) have fewer side-effects, are safer, and better tolerated.

2) Heterocyclics (HCAs). They have fewer side-effects than the tricyclics: amoxapine, maprotiline, bupropion, and trazodone.

The first generation of heterocyclics (HCAs), Amoxapine and Maprotiline, cause neurologic side-effects.

The second generation of heterocyclics are Bupropion (Wellbutrin) and Trazodone (Desyrel). Trazodone has no neurologic side-effects. Buproprion has no side-effects, but may be a stimulant. Their cardiovascular effects are orthostatic hypotension, arrhythmia (sudden death), anticholinergic effects (dry mouth, palpitations, tachycardia, urinary retention, constipation, loss of memory).

Hypotension and tachycardia are the most frequent complications of heterocyclics; tricyclics and heterocyclics can be lethal with overdose. Falls and fractures (hip, skull) are reported. Disturbance in mental functions is frequent, especially in the elderly.

3) Selective Serotonin Reuptake Inhibitors (SSRIs): Fluoxetine (Prozac) which is long acting, Paroxetine (Paxil), and Sertraline (Zoloft).

Fluoxetine (Prozac) was the first, followed by Sertraline and Paroxetin. There is no severe side-effects, but there still can be anorexia, nausea, some anxiety and nervousness. Note delayed onset of action. But effective dose can be given from the beginning. There is wide safety margin and no life-threatening toxic effects.

They are good for prolonged treatment with fewer side-effects than TCA or HCA. They are very popular.

4) Anxiolytics. Unlike the SSRIs they are not recommended for prolonged treatment, but have quicker action. All are benzodiazines (BZDs), except buspirone. They are very popular today.

Some are more anxiolytic, others are more hypnotic (they produce sleep), and others are also sedatives (they relieve pain). Some are short-acting, others long-acting. The side-effects of anxiolytics are sedation and sleep, amnesia, disinhibition (agitation, hostility, anger). The issues of dependence and withdrawal symptoms have been widely emphasized in view of their widespread use.

Anxiolytics are also indicated when psychiatric disorders are present.

In terminal patients with severe pain, a combination of opiates and anxiolytics will be very effective.

The indications for anxiolytics are milder forms of depression, combined anxiety and depression, associated complex medical problems where usual antidepressants (TCA and HCA) are risky to use mostly during the acute phase.

a. BZD anxiolytics: alprazolam (Xanax), clorazepata (Tranxene), diazepam (Valium), lorazepam (Ativan), and chlordiazepoxide (Librium)

b. BZD hypnotics: Flurazepam (Dalmane), Quazepam (Doral), and Triazolam (Halcion).

c. Non-BZD anxiolytics. The most important is buspirone (Buspar). It has no side-effects like BZD, but slow acting.

d. Non-BZD hypnotics: Zopiclone and Zopidem (used in Europe only).

5) Monoamine Oxidase Inhibitors (MAOI). One should stay away from MAOI because like HCA, and more so like TCA, they produce orthostatic hypotension. The main ones are Isocarboxazid, Phenelzine, and Tranylcypromine. MAOI use should be left to the *psychiatrists* because of side-effects, especially when combined with other antidepressants. MAOI are not first-line drugs because of weight gain, potentially fatal interactions, and orthostatic hypotension. But, MAOI are indicated when combined with atypical psychiatric features.

NEUROLEPTICS (OR ANTIPSYCHOTICS):

Terminal patients may develop a psychotic reaction that has to be treated. A psychosis is the inability to differentiate reality from fantasy. The first medications were the phenothiazine antipsychotics, namely, chlorpromazine (Thorazine). The words neuroleptics, phenothiazines, and antipsychotics can be used interchangeably. The major problem is the unreliability of gastric absorption. They are long acting and can be used once a day. Neurological complications are frequent and the medications should be used with caution. There are no dependence or withdrawal symptoms. Combination of any anti-depressant and a neuroleptic appears to be analgesic in cancer patients. Some researchers compare their sedative action to morphine. The main phenothiazines are:

Fluphenazine: very potent analgesic.

Perphenazine: less potent, but good in combination with amitriptyline.

Haloperidol: well tolerated, but possible hypotension.

Chlorprothixine: less analgesic and more a sedative.

Thioridazine: less potent.

Chlorpromazine: can sometimes produce granulocytopenia.

In using neuroleptics for pain management, one should weigh the side-effects such as delayed and permanent dyskinesia. One should start with an antidepressant and add a neuroleptic only when sleep is normalized but the patient is still in pain. In terminal patients, however, long-term neurological complications should not count.

In bipolar or manic-depressive disorders, successful management is with Lithium which is an excellent mood stabilizer. Anxiolytics are also effective in combination with Lithium.

ANTICONVULSANT (OR ANTIEPILEPTICS):

They form a heterogenous group, and four of them have been used in pain management. The main ones are phenytoin (originally diphenylhydantoin), valproic acid, carbamazepine, and clonazepam. There is occasional success in pain treatment. They all have many side-effects, mostly long-term. All anticonvulsants can cause cognitive and behavioral disorders (loss of memory, motor response). The best indication for pain relief is a mixed diagnosis (painful tic, past herpetic neuralgia) or when refractory to other modes of therapy.

ANTIHISTAMINES AND MUSCLE RELAXANTS:

Hydroxyzine can potentiate the action of opiates in view of respiratory depression associated with high doses of opiates. Contrary to the opiates, the analgesic effect of the antihistamines has a ceiling level.

Elderly Patients

The elderly are susceptible to medications because of impaired cardiovascular system, liver, kidneys, and because of central nervous system (CNS) impairment. Usually start with half of adult doses.

The goal should be keeping the elderly patient mentally, physically, and socially active. Too often, medication does the reverse by undertreatment. Elderly patients are either overtreated or undertreated.

The secondary amines (Desipramine, Nortriptyline) are to be used cautiously because of side-effects.

The new generation of HCA (Tradozone, Bupropion) can also be prescribed cautiously. SSRIs have fewer side-effects than HCA. Psychostimulants may be indicated. MOAIs are not recommended. BZDs are for anxiety and for a short time only. Do not prescribe barbiturate or meprobamate for the elderly. Buspirone is indicated for the elderly.

Complications of antidepressants are orthostatic hypotension (fractured hip, skull), tachycardia, constipation, and urinary retention.

Other complications of advanced cancer and/or its treatment have to be addressed. They may be due to the cancer itself or associated with or increased by medications. They have to be addressed separately with specific medications. The most common are vomiting, diarrhea, dyspnea, nausea, incontinence, bed sores, hiccups, anorexia, coughing, insomnia. They make terminal life a nightmare for the patient as well as the entourage and should be corrected separately.

Drug	Therapeutic Dosage Range (mg/day)	Average (Rng) of Elimination Half-Life (Hours)	Potentially Fatal Drug Interactions
Tricyclics			
Amitriptyline (Elavil, Endep)	75-300	24 (16-46)	Antiarrhythmics, MAOI
Desipramine (Norpramin, Pertofrane)	75-300	18 (12-50)	Antiarrhythmics, MAOI
Imipramine (Janimine, Tofranil)	75-300	22 (12-34)	Antiarrhythmics, MAOI
Nortriptyline (Aventyl, Pamelor)	40-200	26 (18-88)	Antiarrhythmics, MAOI
Heterocyclics			
Amoxapine (Asendin)	100-600	10 (8-14)	MAOI
Bupropion (Wellbutrin)	225-450	14 (8-24)	MAOI (possibly)
Maprotiline (Ludiomil)	100-225	43 (27-58)	MAOI
Trazodone (Desyrel)	150-600	8 (4-14)	—
Selective Serotonin Reuptake Inhibitors (SSRIs)			
Fluoxetine (Prozac)	10-40	168 (72-360)	MAOI
Paroxetine (Paxil)	20-50	24 (3-65)	MAOI
Sertraline (Zoloft)	50-150	24 (10-30)	MAOI
Monoamine Oxidase Inhibitors (MAOIs)			For all 3 MAOI: Vasoconstrictors, decongestants, meperidine, and possibly other narcotics
Isocarboxazid (Marplan)	30-50	Unknown	
Phenelzine (Nardil)	45-90	2 (1.5-4.0)	
Tranylcypromine (Parnate)	20-60	2 (1.5-3.0)	

Drug	Anti-cholinergic	Central Nervous System		Cardiovascular		Other	Wt Gn (Over 6 kg)
		Drowsi-ness	Insomnia Agitation	Orthostatic Hypo-tension	Cardiac Arrhyth-mia	Gastro-intestinal Distress	
TCA: Amitriptyline	4+	4+	0	4+	3+	0	4+
Imipramine	3+	3+	1+	4+	3+	1	3+
Desipramine	1+	1	1+	2+	2+	0	1-
Nortriptyline	1+	1+	0	2+	2+	0	1+
HCA Amoxapine	2+	2+	2+	2+	3+	0	1+
Maprotiline	2+	4+	0	0	1+	0	2+
Trazodone	0	4+	0	1+	1+	1+	1+
Bupropion	0	0	2+	0	1+	1+	0
SSRI Fluoxetine	0	0	2+	0	0	3+	0
Paroxetine	0	0	2+	0	0	3+	0
Sertraline	0	0	2+	0	0	3+	0
MAOI: Monoamine oxidase inhibitors	1	1+	2+	2+	0	1+	2+

0 = absent or rare   1+ 2+ = in between   3+4+ = relatively common

Physical symptoms associated with depression that have to be dealt with separately are tachycardia, palpitations, chest tightness; breathing difficulties; nausea, diarrhea, intestinal cramps; dry mouth. Anxiety responds better to anxiolytics (BZD), while panic attacks respond better to antidepressants such as SSRI.

BZDs have fewer side-effects than the TCAs and are just as effective. They are the most widely used, even in some cases on a long-term basis. In large doses, BZDs are euphoric. BZD is commonly prescribed for long-term use in anxiety and insomnia. But BZDs are really not good for long-term treatment. The advantage of BZD is that they act quickly, within the first week of prescription. BZDs act better for short-term prescription and lose effect afterward. In general, first week of treatment is excellent and long-term effects after four months is not documented. Buspirone (non-BZD) takes longer to act and is not good for acute episodes, but is effective when patient no longer responds to BZD.

In summary, acute anxiety is treated with BZD (not beyond 12 weeks), but chronic anxiety is better treated with buspirone. For long-term therapy, SSRI such as Prozac, is better.

Barbiturate and barbiturate-like drugs (chloral hydrate) and also tranquilizers (Miltown, Equanil) are considered less safe than BZD in terms of tolerance, habituation, danger of overdose, and interaction with alcohol.

The most dangerous side-effect of antidepressants is orthostatic hypotension. Anti-depressants do not cause addiction, but they cause withdrawal symptoms with abrupt discontinuation (sleep disturbance with powerful dreams). Discontinuance should be gradual.

Antidepressants can also be used in pain management (Paoli et al., 1960) and are recommended for the treatment of chronic pain.

The relation of pain to depression was studied by Turk et al., (1987) and Getto et al., (1987). Merskey et al., (1972) used them for cancer pain. The studies are extensive in view of interest by psychiatrists (Montilla et al., 1963; McGee and Alexander, 1979; Oliver, 1979; Digregorio and Kozin, 1986). The clinical management of medication has been studied by Fawcett, Scheftner, Clark, et al. (1987).

Always select the drug that also treats another complaint, like poor sleep, for instance.

Inform patients that side-effects do not persist. Long-term use is generally safe and the analgesic effect persists.

Depression almost always can be successfully treated one way or another. When a medication does not work, try one from another class rather than the same class.

Most antidepressant medications have comparable efficacy. No antidepressant medication is clearly more effective than another and no single medication results in remission for all patients. One has to consider (1) short-term versus long-term; (2) prior positive response; (3) associated illnesses; (4) once-a-day dosage; (5) personal experience.

Although one has to watch for side-effects, one should always remember that they are less important in terminal patients and that patients eventually adapt to side-effects.

With coronary disease, drugs such as bupropion or fluoxetine that are not hypotensive or do not produce conductive changes, are preferable.

When there is obsessive compulsive disorder associated with depression, drugs such as fluoxetine (Prozac) show efficacy in both conditions.

Atypical psychiatric features would suggest more MAOI or SSRI than TCA. If there is a possibility of suicide by overdose, prescribe doses for one week only. In this case, heterocyclics (bupropion or trazodone) or SSRI may be preferred.

Be ready to change medication if results are insufficient because it is highly unusual for the patient not to respond to at least one medication. Medication adjustment is simple: since half-life is usually more than 24 hours the best is daily dose at bedtime to minimize the side-effects. One should begin with low dosage (25-50 mg desipramine daily) and increase the dosage every 1-3 weeks until full effect or there are side-effects. The side-effects will decrease in time. Fluoxetine (Prozac) may be started at 20mg daily or less in the morning and increase in only

4-6 weeks. With fluoxetine, some patients may initially become hyperactive or develop insomnia. Use sleep as the target symptom. Increase every few days until sleep is satisfactory. Depending on side-effects, one may increase or decrease the dose. If there is difficulty in swallowing, use liquid form.

Underdosing is a common cause of nonresponse. By six weeks, full, partial, or no response will be seen. Sometimes it takes up to three months to see full effects. If little or no response is observed, consider one of the following options: increase dosage, add, or substitute other medications. Switching medication is often preferred.

Tricyclic, heterocyclic, and SSRI differ considerably in pharmacological action and side-effects. Therefore, it is reasonable to change a standard TRA to a newer medication such as bupropion (HCA), fluoxetine (Prozac, SSRI), paroxetine (Paxil, SSRI), or sertraline (Zoloft, SSRI).

MAOI may be more effective when there is no response to TCA.

There is no evidence that these antidepressive medication dosages should be tapered. Planning its administration for 4-9 months is satisfactory.

The combination of sedative, hypnotic, or anxiolytic agents and antidepressants is to be avoided, at least for the time being, because the pharmacological action of the combination in terminal patients needs to be studied.

In conclusion, selection has to be empirical and revised if necessary.

Most of these medications have not been used for terminal patients but most are approved for depression and for geriatric patients, so that FDA approval for use in terminal patients is not necessary.

There are three kinds of approval: (1) approved indication by FDA; (2) labeled indication by the pharmaceutical company and also approved by FDA; and (3) unlabeled use by the physician beyond package insert. Physicians are free to prescribe a drug based on their clinical experience.

Chapter 18

MOOD ELEVATION: AN ALTERNATIVE TO FEAR, ANXIETY AND DEPRESSION

Come, death, oh beautiful bride. –Cabalist Prayer for the Dead

I am convinced that at least some of us can face death differently, that we can look forward to it and even embrace it euphorically when the time comes. This type of death has already been suggested by Carl Jung's archetype concept and been described when researchers recount near death experiences (NDE). The emotional state I'm referring to transcends simple resignation and acceptance when one is about to die. It is more than the case of a physically sick and handicapped terminal patient looking at death as a way out, with the fear of death slowly fading. It goes beyond feeling as if one has had it with life and that it's trivial activities are no longer meaningful.

What I believe is possible is a meditative state that allows death to be approached peacefully and calmly; these feelings facilitate a transition to euphoria and even ecstasy. This mood elevation may seem unlikely, but I have witnessed it more times than you might imagine. The problem is that dying patients are rarely allowed to express this mood.

BARRIERS TO MOOD ELEVATION

Many conditions and circumstances prevent this mood from being expressed. Perhaps the greatest obstacle is the group surrounding the dying patient—family, friends, physicians, nurses, hospital personnel—as well as societal attitudes. They communicate to the patient that death and dying are tragic events. They create a tremendously somber and fearful mood—a mood that is oppressive in its intensity. To express contentment or euphoria in the midst of this oppressive atmosphere would seem like heresy.

Another barrier is physical pain. If this pain is not relieved, people focus on the organic disease that created the terminal condition.

It is difficult to make peace and express joy when one's body is being wracked with pain. Meditation demands concentration, and it's difficult to concentrate on anything when one is in great pain.

Similarly, this elevated mood won't surface unless depression and anxiety are alleviated. This can be done relatively easily with anti-depressants. Good sleep patterns also are important to establish in this regard. Terminal patients often wake in the middle of the night complaining of pain, depression and anxiety; they then are sleepy and irritable during the day because of this lack of sleep. As a result, it's difficult to feel good about anything.

Another obstacle is isolation. Though it's possible to experience pre-death euphoria when we are alone, it is much easier to experience if we have someone to talk to openly about feelings related to dying and death. It's usually not important who that person is—a spouse, a relative, a friend, a religious figure, a doctor—as long as he or she is willing to discuss the subject as deeply and emotionally as the dying person desires. This open atmosphere makes it much easier to elevate one's mood in the face of death.

It's worth noting that drug addicts dying of AIDS often are nonchalant and sometimes ecstatic as death approaches while homosexuals dying of AIDS usually exhibit anxiety and fear. Though the disease is the same, the drug addict has the advantage of addictive drugs that result in mood-elevation and euphoria.

At this point, let me make a distinction that's important to keep in mind throughout this discussion. Drugs don't produce euphoria as much as they make it possible for it to surface. In other words, the euphoria is natural and resides within all of us; the drugs simply open up a path for it to emerge.

Following is a list of the most common mood elevating drugs. Here, too, I will stress that lay people, more than the medical professionals, are familiar with their beneficial effects. Some of these drugs, i.e., pain relievers, anxiolytics, and mood elevators, have multiple effects.

Morphine is named after Morpheus, the Greek god of dreams. Throughout history, opium has been used to produce euphoria, mood elevation and dreams. As one of the components of opium, morphine is extracted from the juice of poppy (papaver somniferum). The effects of opium were described by the ancient Greeks in the third century BC. It is the drug most written about in medical history, and its advantages, side-effects, toxicity and abuse are well-documented. Sydenham in 1680 called it "a gift of God" to relieve man's sufferings, and today it is still mostly used to relieve physical pain. Because of its abuse and the likelihood of addiction, the main purpose of morphine—to relieve pain and produce euphoria—is often overlooked. People perceive the negatives of the drug to outweigh the positives. We know, however, that opium was used throughout history for the pleasant sensations it produced rather than for analgesia. For many centuries opium has represented in the Orient what cigarettes and alcohol currently represent in the Occident.

Each culture favors one type of mood elevation over others. Certainly our culture favors alcohol and frowns on opium and its derivatives. There's a certain justification to this sentiment, since opium is more addictive than alcohol. But part of the negative connotations of opium has to do with the blaring anti-drug messages our society sends out. These messages make it difficult to look at opium and morphine objectively and see the positives along with the negatives. When it comes to mood elevation, however, no drug has proved to be more effective than opium and its purified extracts or similar derivatives. To smoke a pipe of opium, hashish, or cannabis once or twice a week has been and still is a common practice in many parts of the world, just as common as an evening cocktail or glass of wine is in our culture. These smoking habits do not lead to any serious addictions. At most, they lead to habituation and can usually be given up without much difficulty. The use of opium extracts, such as morphine or heroin, lead to addiction.

Morphine is difficult to synthesize, and it is less expensive to extract from the poppy. The usual therapeutic dose is 10mg. The main morphine derivatives, the semi-synthetics, and synthetic similar drugs are all mood elevators and include:

1. Heroin (diacetylmorphine or diamorphine) is not used in the United States. It is the most powerful morphine derivative and quickly leads to drug addiction when overused. It certainly is a potent mood elevator, and this use deserves more study. Unfortunately, this use is known more by drug addicts than by the medical professionals.

2. Dilaudid (hydromorphine, 5mg, ½ dose of morphine), it can be taken by mouth or suppository. It is the most commonly prescribed drug for patients outside a hospital confinement because of its easy titration.

3. Demerol (Meperidine or pethidine), 75mg, can be taken orally or through injection. It is most frequently used in hospitals to calm patients before surgery or to relieve pain after surgery. Its pharmacology is best known by anesthesiologists. Very few patients realize that Demerol is a morphine derivative.

4. Fentanyl, 0.1mg, can be used in suppository form. This is an important drug because it can be used when patients are vomiting or have sores over their body, and other modes of administration are difficult or impossible.

5. Methadone, 10mg, can be taken orally. This drug is gaining more and more importance because it is a good mood elevator and is minimally addictive. It is good for long-term usage, and as a substitute for drug addiction.

6. Codeine (methylmorphine), 30mg, can be taken orally, and is the most benign morphine derivative. It is the best drug to start with for pain relief and mood elevation.

7. Darvon, 65mg, can be taken orally and Talwin, 50mg, can be taken orally. These two drugs are prescribed for outpatients and are excellent in the stages when pain is mild and anxiety is minimal. They quickly reestablish peace of mind.

Morphine and derivatives produce analgesia and mood elevation without loss of consciousness. Morphine relieves not only physical pain but also the affective response associated with physical pain, anxiety, fear and panic. The mechanism by which opioids produce euphoria, tranquillity and mood elevation is not entirely clear. Most likely, euphoria spontaneously appears when physical pain and anxiety are relieved.

When abused and overused, these drugs may lead to mild or serious complications and medical supervision is always necessary. The main side-effect of opioids is respiratory depression. Deaths from morphine overdose are always due to respiratory arrest. The triad indicative of morphine poisoning is depressed respiration, coma and pinpoint pupils. Naloxone is the typical opioid antagonist.

The other main side-effects after extended use are constipation, urinary retention, nausea, vomiting, and dizziness. The duration of analgesia increases with age, but the sedation effect for a given dose does not change.

Keep in mind that opioids not only relieve physical pain but also impact the emotions associated with pain. The emotional and social repercussions of physical pain should not be taken lightly; the barriers to euphoria that they erect are as real as the pain. In cancer patients, opioids produce not only analgesia but also mental tranquillity, elation and exhilaration.

One can diminish the dose of morphine and maintain the same effects by combining it with amphetamines (Dexedrine) and/or NSAIDs (see Chapter 17).

Steroids offer a mild euphoria, increased appetite, and a sense of well-being. These advantages definitely outweigh the risks. However, one has to watch for preexisting conditions such as psychiatric disorders, active infections or gastrointestinal disturbances.

COCAINE

Smoking cocoa leaves is common in many parts of the world, and it rarely leads to tolerance and dependence. The desired effect is mood elevation and euphoria, but few scientific studies exist related to this effect.

Cocaine is a naturally occurring alkaloid found in the leaves of

Erythroxylon coca. It is used as a local anesthetic agent (1 to 10% solution) on the mucous membranes of the oral, nasal, and laryngeal cavities but not the eye because of corneal toxicity. Rapid and excessive absorption through the mucous membranes may lead to adverse effects characterized by nervousness, but also a feeling of well being and euphoria. Hallucinations (visual, auditory, tactile, olfactory, gustatory) also can occur.

Small intravenous (IV) doses of cocaine may produce bradycardia, moderate (20mg) dose will produce tachycardia, but large IV doses (1 to 2gm) will lead to sudden death by respiratory failure. Repeated topical application may lead to tolerance and dependence. The drug can be abused through intranasal application.

MARIJUANA

Marijuana (hashish in the Middle East and Northern Africa), also known as grass or pot, comes from the flowering tops of hemp plants. It is by far the most commonly used illicit drug in the United States with half of the young adults experiencing or having experienced it. Most commonly the plant is cut, dried, chopped and incorporated into cigarettes. Smoking a cigarette or 20mg of cannabinol (the active component extracted from marijuana) produces euphoria, a sense of well being combined with a feeling of relaxation. There is sleepiness when alone or laughter with interaction. This is contrary to LSD (see next paragraph) which produces a state of heightened wakefulness. In addition, there is also confusion, unreality, depersonalization or what is called temporal disintegration and an amotivational syndrome. This lasts 4-8 hours. The half-time duration is 30 hours but metabolites can be detected in urine for several weeks. Experienced users can get more effects from smoking marijuana than beginners. Withdrawal symptoms are mild.

Marijuana is benign enough so that its use is legal (although carefully regulated) in some states. Its main component (cannabinol) can be prescribed by doctors under specific conditions. This happens rarely, though, because the medical profession is not familiar with its use, and fear of addiction is widespread.

These drugs are the most frequently used mood elevators, although, again, lay people are more familiar with them than the medical professionals.

Drugs that induce psychedelic effects have been used for centuries. The peyote cactus (containing mescaline) and mushrooms (containing psilocin) were used in America before the Spanish conquest. In the 1950s, hundreds of scientific articles were written on LSD in regard to self-exploration. LSD is easy to manufacture synthetically.

The most common psychedelic drugs, lysergic acid diethylmide (LSD), mescaline, and psilocin, are easily accessible, although illegal. They produce a heightened sense of clarity, increased self-esteem and also the feeling of being a passive observer—a spectator ego rather than an active and directing force. In a way, there is heightened cognitive awareness, though there is argument about what this awareness entails. There is also a diminished capacity to differentiate the boundaries of one object from another and self from the environment. The line between unreality and reality often blurs. This LSD-like effect is completely different from the amphetamine-like effect of very meaningful and directed overactivity. Some psychedelics may even produce ecstasy.

In man, oral doses of LSD, such as 20 to 25 mcg produce central nervous system (CNS) effects in sensitive individuals.

Doses of 1 microgram/kg of body weight leads to euphoria, visual illusions, affective symptoms. Overlapping of sensory perception still occurs. Synesthesia, or overflow from one sensory modality to another, is common: colors are heard and sounds are seen. Subjective time is seriously altered and seems to pass very slowly. There is loss of boundaries between the self and the environment. This is called a trip by users and thoughts and memories can emerge. There may be gaiety and elation or the opposite, such as distress, depression and fear. There is a sense of detachment and the conviction that one is magically in control.

The half-life is three hours and the entire syndrome is cleared within 12 hours. LSD is 100 times more potent than psilocin and 4000 times more than mescaline. Psilocin is called the Mexican magic mushroom. Students call it the recreational drug. It was used by psychiatrists to facilitate psychotherapy. It has psychedelic and amphetamine-like properties. LSD was proposed as an adjunct to psychotherapy and for the treatment of alcoholism and drug addiction.

There appears to be no striking increase in genetic abnormality or congenital malformation among American tribes that have used mescaline for several generations. Side-effects are not uncommon, however, and are called bad trips with depression, anxiety and panic.

Flashback or recurrent drug effects without the drug are a puzzling phenomenon. They occur in more than 15% of users and occur up to several years after last LSD exposure.

Psychedelic drugs are well-known from a pharmacological point of view, but they have rarely been tested on terminal patients. They should be more widely used on terminal patients, at least as a first trial. I have seen few terminal patients who died in a state of euphoria with the use of LSD. Psychedelic drugs are not addictive in the serious sense of the word. They lead at most to habituation and most people eventually give it up. The fear of addiction to these drugs is markedly exaggerated.

ADJUVANT DRUGS

Benzodiazepines (mainly Librium and Valium, but also Librax, Tranxene, Dalmane, Alivan, Doral, Halcion, etc.), are mostly used for acute rather than chronic conditions. They are sedative, anxiolytic, and hypnotic. They are postulated to produce disinhibition (or previously suppressed response). They are used mostly to treat anxiety, insomnia, and panic. These drugs are mostly used for short term, but long-term use has not been evaluated. They facilitate euphoria and mood elevation.

Antidepressants (mostly SSRI, such as Prozac) and anxiolytics (such as Valium and Librium) will work indirectly on mood elevation. All antidepressants are euphoric in high doses. They also produce disinhibition.

My experience is that these drugs are more frequently used by the surrounding family than by terminal patients. The two indications are not mutually exclusive and they should be prescribed to both parties under proper medical supervision.

Music therapy (Gregorian chant) is a recent, non-drug addition in this category. It is mostly indicated for terminal patients who prefer isolation. It will easily reinforce the euphoric effect of previous drugs. Individual hearing systems can easily be supplied to patients who appear to benefit from the system.

A RATIONALE FOR MOOD ELEVATING DRUGS

Once pain and depression have been relieved, any one or combination of these drugs should be considered for use with terminal patients. They can produce a calm and accepting attitude toward dying and death as well as a euphoric state. I have seen patients treated this way who are serious, relaxed, and enjoy complete peace of mind as death draws near. I have also seen patients welcoming death with exuberance and opposing any attempt to stop the dying process. As astonishing as it may seem, some of them were smiling, laughing and even joking as death approached.

While all these feelings occur naturally, they rarely are allowed to do so because of all the reasons I've discussed throughout this book. To recreate these natural feelings, we can use the drugs that have emerged from the tremendous progress and diversity in pharmacology today.

Philosophically, I'm convinced that the death experience is something we must live through; it is not only a necessary part of life but a meaningful and potentially ecstatic phase of our existence. Most of us, unfortunately, are deprived of this experience and future generations will probably benefit from what we're learning about death and dying today.

Given the possibility of a positive, meaningful death, it's a mystery why anyone allows other people to interfere and turn dying into a fearful, extremely depressing experience. Perhaps the concept of an ecstatic death is so foreign to what we understand death to be that it seems bizarre and scary. Perhaps we naturally choose what is familiar to us rather than an option that appears to be ill-defined and uncertain. The only real definition of the drug-assisted dying process I'm proposing comes from people who have related their Near Death Experiences. These people have had a taste of the euphoria that can accompany life as it's slipping away, and it is something worth trying to duplicate in people who are really dying.

At the moment, however, this is an ambitious goal. For most people, dying and death are dominated by fear. This is not a natural reaction but one spawned by the way we manage the dying process. Mood elevating drugs provide us with hope of a better, more natural path.

Why Doctors Don't Do Anything

Although all the necessary tools and all the necessary knowledge are at hand, there is no organized system for doctors to apply this science. Instead, there's a disorganized system made up of isolated initiatives, sidetracked initiatives and counter-initiatives. In addition, doctors are paralyzed by apathy and inertia, a nothing-you-can-do-about-it attitude.

The medical profession has to create a new specialty for dealing with terminal patients and determine in a scientific way which drugs work best for which people. This will depend on many factors such as age, past medical history, current disease and health conditions, personality, state of mind. Anxious people will be treated one way; depressed people another. Some people may be satisfied with music therapy; other will need a continuous drip of intravenous morphine.

Very few doctors will volunteer for this type of role. I understand their reluctance, and it reminds me of what is happening in the area of abortion. Abortions on request are legal today, but prejudices against abortionists remain. Today, it is more and more difficult for hospitals to recruit doctors willing to perform abortions and those who perform them keep it a secret as if they were ashamed of it. A doctor who happens to commit a serious mistake in treating any patient will probably be excused for it. But, if a doctor commits a serious mistake in performing an abortion, God help him, because his medical license will be revoked and he may even wind up in jail. It's understandable why doctors don't like to perform abortions, and it's also understandable why doctors wouldn't want to specialize in treating dying patients, easing their coming death, and sometimes shortening the terminal state. Should a doctor overtreat a patient and precipitate death, or should a patient be wrongly diagnosed as terminal and end up dying as a result of drug treatment, the responsible doctor would be in serious trouble. Also, the fear of producing drug addiction and of these drugs falling into the hands of drug addicts make most doctors turn away from this new specialty.

It's also true that doctors often reject any approach to death that isn't firmly grounded in reality and practicality. For them, death is the enemy, and that's all there is to it. From an historical point of view, medicine had a hard time separating itself from witchcraft and from religion, and doctors would be reluctant to return to what they would consider an unscientific approach to terminal patients.

At the same time, only doctors have the knowledge and training to do the job. They are the only ones with the skills to do the research, to compile statistics for each every available drug and the indications and contraindications of each drug, and to do the follow-up for positive or negative results.

Still, resistance to developing a system of drug protocols for dying patients is significant, as the following anecdote attests. Recently, I attended a conference of anesthesiologists. The subject was about preoperative medication. Discussions centered on the dosage and effect of Demerol and barbiturates administered to patients before surgery in order to get patients completely relaxed prior to anesthesia. At the end of the presentation, during the question and answer period, I stood up and asked the following question: What is the dose of Demerol and/or barbiturate that could result in the death of the patient when administered through an intravenous line? I tried to present this question as innocently as possible, giving the reason for my question that I wanted to know what dosage limits I should stay away from. But the reaction I produced among these anesthesiologists was a horror. One anesthesiologist thought I wanted to terminate the life of a dying patient, another thought that I wanted to commit suicide. Others protested that they never use drugs for that purpose. When I persisted in my question, most of the members said they did not know the answer, and finally the chairman of the conference told me that he would consult the literature and shortly give me an answer. I am still waiting for him to call me. Of all the different medical specialities, anesthesiologists possess the proper knowledge and tools to help terminal patients find the right type and dosage of drugs, yet they showed no interest in exploring this topic.

Chapter 19

FROM ASSISTED SUICIDE AND MERCY KILLING TO ASSISTED TERMINAL CONDITION (ATC)

"Thou Shalt Not Kill" —6th Commandment

The media has done many stories on this topic because of Dr. Jack Kevorkian's crusade and because the subject is inherently controversial. Assisted suicide and mercy killings have legal and ethical implications that are hotly debated, and it's relatively easy to make a convincing argument for either side of the issue. People become very worked up arguing both pro and con.

I'd like to take a somewhat different perspective on the topic in this chapter. The phrase, right to die , shapes this perspective. It is a right that is often denied to terminal patients; they are not allowed to die prematurely, and they are kept alive in terrible pain and with mounting fear until a natural death occurs. Should we have a right to die when we want or must we wait until technology and medications can no longer sustain our lives? To answer these questions, let's begin by placing them in a broader context.

A Brief History of Homicide

We have always killed and death has always been feared and painful. Intervention in the natural order of things by brutally murdering another person is a theme throughout the history of mankind and inherited from our animal ancestry. Animals kill each other for the purpose of eating each other, to defend themselves and to protect their progeny, their females or their territory. Humans also kill each other to defend or take each other's possessions. Human societies, however, became possible only when the right to kill was regulated. With hindsight, some of these regulations appear barbaric: mothers could kill newborns if they could not support them or men could kill their wives for infidelity. Other regulations included rules of war, capital punishment and so on.

Jesus Christ was the first in human history to take a firm stand against any form of killing, and Christianity has adhered to this stance. Even during the Middle Ages and afterward when the death penalty was imposed for any heretical deviation, the Church never carried out any executions (a lay person was always assigned this task). With the French Revolution and the Enlightenment that followed, the death penalty was debated, done away with and restored many times. While capital punishment today is less common throughout the world, we still have written and unwritten regulations about what justifies capital punishment. Killing a child or a pregnant woman is never forgiven. Murders of passion often result in less severe sentences and sometimes recommendations for psychiatric treatment rather than jail.

This brief history should give you a sense that we've always been willing to end a life prematurely as punishment, in anger, for the purposes of vengeance and so on. Just as we interfere with other laws of nature, we interfere with natural death and it's a very human thing to do. Keep this fact in mind as we look at some of the following right to die issues.

DRUG USE VERSUS DRUG ABUSE

Unlike the animalistic and brutal forms of killing practiced throughout history, drug-induced death is relatively peaceful and painless. At the beginning of the century, pharmacology made tremendous progress extracting opiates from plants and synthesizing barbiturates. Analgesia (relief of pain) and anesthesia (artificial sleep) opened doors to more complex surgery. Further progress was made as medications were administered in more effective ways for given conditions, taken by mouth, injection (intramuscular, subcutaneous, intravenous) or inhaled.

An unfortunate consequence of these pharmacological advances was drug addiction. People began taking these drugs to relieve anxiety and boredom as well as for pure recreational use. Not only did people begin dying from drug overdoses, but a huge, illegal industry was born that is marked by greed, gangs and violence. Because of all the media coverage of drug overdoses and the deaths caused directly and indirectly by drug trafficking, it's difficult to gain acceptance for medical use of narcotics—especially heroin.

At the same time, most people are unaware that these drugs are unsurpassed when it comes to relieving pain and anxiety; that they can produce euphoric effects even in those who are dying; and that they can put people to sleep (temporarily or permanently) humanely. The medical community restricts use of these barbiturates to acute and short-term conditions and would never prescribe them for chronic, long-term conditions for fear of creating drug dependency. They also restrict information about the benefits of these drugs, especially for terminal patients.

Certainly the chronic use of barbiturates is risky because the dangerous levels that could lead to coma and even death stay the same even after prolonged use while the dosage needed to produce the desired effect increases. At the same time, however, this risk is largely irrelevant when we're talking about treatment for terminal patients. Not only could these drugs be used for assisted suicide, but they also could be used to relieve all the previously described symptoms associated with the process of dying. To see terminal patients who are terribly fearful or in great pain and know that they could be dying pain-free, anxiety-free and euphoric is devastating. We possess the pharmaceutical tools to make dying and death a much more sane and humane experience, and we're not taking full advantage of them.

Assisted Suicide and Mercy Killing

Non-pharmaceutical modes of suicide (hanging, shooting, stabbing, jumping out of a window or off a bridge) were so awful to contemplate and painful to carry out that they weren't a viable option for many terminal patients. Drugs, on the other hand, provide a much more acceptable alternative for these patients; it is the equivalent of being put to sleep. I have been put to sleep by an anesthesiologist for minor surgery, and I can assure anyone that being put to sleep by injection is like a dream, and when properly administered pain or anxiety are absent.

Assisted suicide can be a complicated subject and often requires an expert assistant. To avoid any legal implications, the assistant refrains from direct participation in the act: he supplies the necessary equipment (or tells you how to obtain it); he supplies the drugs (or prescribes them and the candidate for suicide buys them from the pharmacy) and instructs on proper usage.

Another form of assisted suicide involves giving a patient a simple prescription for barbiturates with the instruction to take only one pill at bedtime. Doctors tell patients that to take more than one pill a day would be dangerous or even fatal. The patient goes home and takes all the pills in the bottle. I do not know how many of my colleagues are voluntarily or involuntarily involved in this type of assisted suicide, but I suspect there are more than a few. I even knew a hospitalized patient who put aside the sleeping pill given to her at bedtime by the nurse. The nurses are always instructed to make sure the patient swallows the medication in their presence, but this patient put it under her tongue and took it out of her mouth after the nurse walked away. When she was discharged after two weeks, she had accumulated enough medication to kill herself.

Many terminal patients are too weak to carry out these procedures themselves, even when given the proper instructions for assisted suicide. In those cases, mercy killing becomes necessary. The majority of the medical profession remains neutral on this subject, meaning they will not make any recommendations but will follow any legal directives. Others are vociferously against mercy killing, convinced that life should be extended under any circumstances and at any cost.

MORE THAN JUST SEMANTICS

The terms, assisted suicide and mercy killing, are really misnomers. While the terminology may not seem important on the surface, it has a tremendous impact on how we frame the issues involved.

Assisted suicide, for instance, is light years removed from other forms of suicide. Typically, people who kill themselves are young and in good health but depressed over the loss of a job, the end of a romantic relationship or some other life issue. While there are often other factors that create the conditions for someone to commit suicide, the majority of these people have a choice. If they chose not to kill themselves, the odds are that they would live for many more years in good physical health. A dying patient, on the other hand, doesn't have much of a choice; she's living under a death sentence and is often bedridden, severely incapacitated and suffering from a painful disease.

Perhaps more significantly, the terminal patient who kills himself has thought long and hard about what he is going to do and accepted the fact that one way or another, death is close at hand. He is simply moving from near-death to death, and he wants to make the transition less emotionally and physically painful. By using available technology and drugs, this person is revolting against extending a life that is no longer worth living.

In our society, suicide is a pejorative term, and it scares people away. There are also certain religious prohibitions against suicide. No one wants to be the subject of gossip where people at the funeral whisper, "He committed suicide," or "He took an overdose." It suggests the dying person was a coward because he refused to fight death to the bitter end. It suggests that terminal patients have a real choice; that if they fight hard enough, they might triumph over death. This is of course an absurd notion and assisted suicide is an absurd term. What is really happening is that this person is accelerating the dying process by days or weeks and making it less painful.

Mercy killing is an equally inaccurate term, in that no one is being killed. Killing or murder suggests that someone willfully and wantonly takes the life of another; that the person who is killed wanted to live and was unfairly deprived of a potentially wonderful life. When doctors or nurses speed the death of a patient in terrible pain or in a coma from which they'll never wake, they are doing nothing that resembles killing, at least in the sense that society thinks about that word. The adjective, mercy, doesn't soften the phrase much; it still sounds like a terrible thing to do to someone. Perhaps we would come up with a new term if the process were refined. Once the patient has given the proper consent and all legal requirements have been met, an intravenous line could be inserted and when the patient is falling asleep on his own, the medication could be injected into the vein and the patient would not wake up. This more natural method might give rise to a more acceptable descriptive terms. I propose a new denomination: Assisted Terminal Condition (ATC). This new term does not appear repulsive.

We automatically associate death with pain, anxiety, and dread, failing to recognize that modern drugs can induce death painlessly, without anxiety and with mood elevation and even euphoria. If people understood that these drugs could make death easier, then death might have different connotations. Unfortunately, the substance abuse problem has been used as an excuse to deprive dying patients of badly needed drugs.

Of course, these drugs are very powerful and require expert administration. For instance, a dose of 100mg of morphine or any of its derivatives, or 50mg of barbiturates taken by subcutaneous injection, by mouth, by suppository, or slowly through an intravenous line, would lead to a painless death. But there could be problems: medication allergies or intolerance, bad reaction, drug hypersensitivity, unexpected change of patient's mood, patient vomiting, and so on. Only qualified physicians can handle these problems and when people without expertise try to administer these drugs, unexpected complications occur. Presently, only isolated physicians (Dr. Kevorkian, for instance) have developed expertise and for the time being this expertise is not generally available to the medical profession.

Helping people die requires a highly organized process. A complete medical profile is necessary to evaluate the health of the patient. A psychological evaluation by a psychiatrist, psychologist, or social worker is necessary to thoroughly appraise the state of mind of the candidate for death and make sure it fits the outlined criteria. Finally, special committees made up of representatives from different agencies should give final clearance. Assisted terminal condition (ATC) is the death of the future.

The only country that has a system like this is Holland, and their approach should serve as a guide to other countries.

How Other Countries Handle These Issues

Attitudes toward the right-to-die movement vary according to countries and cultures. Judeo-Christian and Islamic cultures essentially reject the idea of suicide, assisted suicide and mercy killing. Many cultures consider the termination of life as a private matter; they believe dying to be nothing more than a passage from one form of existence to another, albeit a serious passage with sacred rituals. On the contrary, many Eastern cultures are convinced that dying is a transit to Heaven, and any interference with it is highly sacrilegious.

In Africa, some people believe all life is only a part of the surrounding universe and death is considered nothing more than a return to Mother Earth.

In Eskimo and American Indian cultures, life is considered a struggle to stay alive and when one is no longer capable of struggling, one is considered figuratively dead. In these circumstances, you're expected to hasten death and surrounding family and friends will oblige by giving you a helping hand. Similar practices are found in the Polynesian Islands.

Japanese culture, although not democratic until recently, has always recognized the right to suicide (*hara-kiri*). There are other democratic cultures besides ours, however, that view suicide in almost criminal terms.

Not too many countries have taken a stand on terminal patients' right to end their lives. Legislation on the subject is rare and covert tolerance is common. In spite of threat of legal action, no one (doctors, nurses, spouses, friends) is condemned for these murders in most countries, providing it can be proved that the motive was to relieve the pain and suffering of a terminal patient.

British legislation has undergone numerous debates. They've examined the medical, religious and political aspects and didn't come to any decision except to recommend that mercy killing and similar procedures are not really murder.

In this country, the patient has the right to refuse any treatment that may extend life, has the right to DNR (do not resuscitate) orders and the family has the right to end life support by pulling the plug in case of brain death. Living wills, a vehicle to delegate that decision if one becomes incompetent, are becoming common practice.

Not allowing death to come naturally and peacefully and creating an artificial, painful, useless, and undesired terminal life with the use of modern technology is considered cruel in many countries. The right to suicide for a dying patient has been established in many countries in Europe (e.g. Holland). Here, Oregon has proposed legislation granting the right of assisted suicide and Washington and New York states are considering guaranteeing any competent person with six months or less to live the right to seek assistance in terminating their life. The Oregon proposed law represents tremendous progress, but it really obliges the patient to commit suicide by administering his own medication. Unfortunately, this maintains the old negative connotation of suicide. In Europe where mercy killing is allowed, the terminal medication does not have to be self-administered.

The Ironies

The first irony is that we live in a society that grants tremendous individual freedoms to its citizens but refuses to grant them the right to die.

The ironic situation in this country is fostered, in part, by many institutions or systems (religious authorities, legal and medical professions, Pro-Life or Pro-Choice groups and political representatives) that claim the right to interfere in any decision impacting the life of these patients. For instance, some organizations claim that we were given the gift of life, and we have to respect and protect it; we are its guardians, and we have no right to dispose of it.

The other irony is that healthy people can terminate their lives any way they wish; they can kill themselves by shooting, hanging, taking an overdose and so on. An incapacitated and handicapped dying patient, however, is unable to commit suicide even though he is in terrible physical pain and emotional agony. Sometimes they can't kill themselves because they're too weak. Other times, they're so fearful and confused that they can't do it themselves. What we've really ended up doing is giving the right to die to healthy people who don't need it and taken it away from unhealthy people who may require it.

Parallels Between Abortion and the Right to Die

Recently I attended a conference on "Suicide in the Elderly: Its Causes and Prevention." The speaker commented at length on this subject, describing the variations demographically, by age, social status, associated medical conditions and so on. He gave the audience a long list of what he believed to be the causes of suicide and then went on to describe its management and prevention. At the end of the presentation, during the question and answer period, I asked the following question: "The Ninth Circuit Court, which governs the westernmost United States, has just established a new constitutional right, namely that all competent persons having six months or less to live are guaranteed the right to arrange for a doctor to help them terminate their lives. If an elderly patient has in hand a medical statement declaring that he has six months to live, are we breaking the law by interfering with any suicide attempt?"

He answered that any desire to die, regardless of age or medical circumstances, indicates a severe mental disturbance in need of immediate medical intervention. I did not push the conversation further or explain that at least in the western United States, any physician who successfully interferes with a legal suicide is exposing himself to medical malpractice for the suffering imposed on a patient who wishes to die but is prevented from doing so.

I did not push the discussion further because I knew the speaker was preaching to the choir. The audience was composed of doctors, psychiatrists, psychologists, psychiatric nurses, general nurses and hospital administrators. From my years of experience working with these people, I knew an overwhelming percentage of them viewed their job as fighting death and extending life no matter what the cost. They were zealous in this belief, and while their zeal to help their patients might be noble, it is also misplaced. If I were to offer an alternative interpretation of how suicide and the elderly should be viewed, I would have been perceived as a heretic. I would have been seen as threatening not only how they saw themselves but also their profession.

For many days, I wondered why everyone was convinced that there was something abnormal about an elderly or terminal patient wanting to die. Then I grasped the similarity between this conference and one I had attended about 20 years ago. The subject revolved around prevention of criminal abortion among women. At that time, to induce an abortion was considered a serious crime. Medical teachings, ethics, religious groups and social norms branded induced abortions a horror and ostracized any doctor involved in an abortion. I remember a colleague of mine who used to report to the police any patient who approached him with an abortion request.

At that time, the speaker on abortion, just like the present speaker on Suicide in the Elderly, presented an analytical study with a long list of pathological conditions that lead women to seek abortions, and then suggested ideas for the management and prevention of abortion. During this talk, the speaker noted that someone who underwent a second abortion needed psychological testing and her actions required further investigation.

The environment has changed a great deal since then. A woman seeking an abortion is no longer considered mentally disturbed. Although abortion on demand is still a hotly debated concept, it has become commonplace throughout the world (though I sometimes wonder if this right has been abused). Unfortunately, we're not similarly enlightened about the right to die. The parallels between the two rights are instructive. Much of our society still views the right to die the way people viewed abortion years ago. We need to be educated about death, and then perhaps our thinking won't be shackled by myths and misconceptions.

We look at death in completely negative terms. When the subject comes up, it triggers a conditioned reflex of repulsion. Automatically, we reject the notion of assisted suicide and an individual's right to die when he wants by whatever means he chooses. Any medical procedure that could hasten death, even if it makes it easier, is completely out of the question. There may be mercy killing for animals, but not for humans. Death has never been integrated into human culture, except in a negative way. To look forward to death and embrace is thought of as abnormal. I understood the speaker on "Suicide in the Elderly" very well when he said he considered it a pathological condition in need of thorough treatment.

This leaves humans with a choice: Either keep on dying in a frightening, painful, unwanted way as determined by history and culture or make a tabula rasa of inherited concepts. If we choose the latter, we can capitalize on progress made in different scientific fields and try to determine new, better conditions for dying. This is easier said than done. To face a new way of death, at variance or even in opposition to inherited and accepted concepts, is frightening. I understand why people want to die the old way.

Contributing to this desire to die the way we've always died is that the desire to live longer and enjoy life today is intense. Life is so good, we don't want to even think about (let alone talk about) how we die. To discuss and determine how one would like to die is almost never approached and, when the time to die comes, the dying person is unable or not allowed to make any decisions. Again, this is part of our tradition and makes it impossible for people to contemplate right-to-die issues in their own lives.

Fear plays a significant role in helping us ignore this subject. People are very reluctant to delegate to others through a Living Will any decision about how their way of dying should be determined. They're so scared of dealing with the issue of their own mortality that they ignore it when they're healthy and lucid. By the time they're ready to deal with it, they're unhealthy and their thinking is muddled.

Beyond this fear, we face other obstacles to reconsidering the right to die issue, including the scary terminology of assisted suicide and mercy killing, instead of a more benign terminology such as Assisted Terminal Condition (ATC). Perhaps just as relevant, we're up against historical patterns and cultural traditions. To look at death differently requires significant changes, and most of us resist change in every area of our lives.

A PHILOSOPHICAL AND LEGAL QUESTION

They Shoot Horses, Don't They? was a popular film about the Great Depression. In this film, a young woman experiencing worsening financial woes decided she was not interested in living any more. She did not have the courage to kill herself and asked a friend to do it for her, and he obliged. He never understood why he was accused of murder. He maintained she did not want to live, she was not fit to live, he did her a great favor by shooting her and was obligated as a friend to kill her since she was too weak to do it herself. He claimed it was mercy killing to shoot a wounded horse that could no longer function, and it was also mercy killing to shoot a human being who could no longer function and wanted to die. The questions raised by this story are these:

Do we own our life and can we dispose of it as we wish?

Assuming we are not allowed to dispose of our life when healthy, do we have that right when we are sick, terminally ill, and suffering?

Do we have the right to delegate this terminal act to someone else and, if we do delegate that right, are those who do it for us murderers?

These are all difficult questions without easy answers. Philosophy, ethics and legal points all complicate our search for the answers. Religious beliefs can add to the confusing mix. The important thing, however, is not to ignore the subject out of fear. We will never make progress and learn to die in ways that a life well-lived deserves until we begin thinking and talking about right-to-die issues. The first step, I believe, is to stop talking about assisted suicide or mercy killing and consider assisted terminal condition. This change of words is more than semantic. It supposes a completely new approach.

Chapter 20

HOPE FOR THE FUTURE

"Nothing has been more intolerable to man than freedom. It is a world filled with uncertainty, fear, and anxiety." —Dostoevsky

Over the years, various cultures and individuals have approached death in a wide variety of ways. While some of these approaches have become traditional and others have faded away, none of them has proven satisfactory. We're still searching for a meaningful, satisfying way to deal with death both on individual and societal levels.

Unfortunately, our search has become troublesome. The trouble begins because some people strongly believe that everyone should enjoy life to the very end because they fully intend to do so (and perhaps they have had friends or family members who have done so). The trouble becomes worse when physically healthy people feel threatened because others who are suffering want to end their lives (rather than have an extended life imposed upon them). The trouble really arrives when those who are enjoying their lives interfere with those who want to end their own lives; they consider them pathological and in need of help.

Healthy people impose rules and extend the lives of those who want to die for a variety of religious or ethical reasons; they also do so because of their fear of death. The challenge for our society and each and every member of it is to move past these reasons and recognize that they stand in the way of a new approach to death and dying.

Courage to Capitalize on our Freedom

To help meet this challenge, we need to keep the following principles or truisms in mind.

1. There is no natural way of dying. Nature, God, or whatever entity one believes in, did not prescribe a specific way to die. While death is natural, there is no natural way in which our life ends. What feels right and meaningful for one person may seem uncomfortable and irrelevant for another.

2. Throughout prehistory and history, all modes of death emanate from cultural imperatives and nothing else. In other words, there's nothing sacred or magical about the various traditions and customs associated with death. They simply seem sacred and magical because they've been handed down from one generation to the next and gained power because they've been the status quo for so long.

3. Our taboos and rituals regarding death are made by the living to accommodate the needs of the living (rather than the needs of the dying). The living are often motivated by different feels and desires than those who are dying. Specifically, the living may be attempting to relieve their own fears about death when they interfere with how someone is dying; the latter have little say in this matter.

4. Dying people should control the process of dying for their own satisfaction and no one else's. It is the responsibility of each person to do inner soul searching and work on how he would like his death handled. Everyone should enjoy complete freedom in this regard and be allowed to script his own death, using whatever technology and science has to offer. Each person should have the choice between a traditional method of dying and various alternatives.

The problem with following these principles is that they grant people a terrifying measure of freedom. Or as Dostoevsky said: Nothing has been more intolerable to man than freedom. It is a world filled with uncertainty, fear, and anxiety. During the Roman Empire, slaves preferred and found it safer to belong to a good master than to have uncertain freedom. Give me freedom or give me death is a popular saying but not a deeply-held belief. Just as there is hierarchy in the animal world, humans still gravitate toward having rules imposed on them. By subordinating ourselves to the rule of others, we don't have to make decisions or endure the burdensome weight of authority. To be free requires a certain amount of courage and a willingness to take risks. At the time of dying, our fear is at its zenith and we are tempted to forsake our freedom and fall back on tradition. No matter how terrible it might be to extend our misery for weeks or months, we choose this option because it is familiar and accepted. It is difficult to muster up the courage to choose a less traditional or accepted alternative. Surrounding people usually don't advocate an innovative approach to death; they too opt for the safe choice.

The only way out of playing it safe is for each of us to search our souls and realize the misery of dying in our culture; that it is not just something that happens to others but to all of us; that we have to think about these matters when we're healthy and have the courage and freedom to contemplate other, better ways of dying.

This doesn't mean that I believe that the result of this contemplation will be for everyone to choose assisted suicide. I'm not advocating any single approach to death. What I am advocating is opening our minds to other possibilities. To talk about this issue in the same terms as we do the abortion issue—to label someone pro-choice or to say that we're interfering with a natural process—is to miss the point. We've always interfered with death; our traditions are simply a result of that interference. What I'm arguing for is that we shouldn't be bound by tradition. I'm suggesting that the mainstream approach to dying is disorganized, irrational, misguided, and cruel and that we need to find a way that is more organized, rational, and purposeful.

IDEAL MODE OF DEATH

Let us imagine what death might be like if nature or some other higher power were guiding this process. Just as we talk about the miracle of life, we could also talk about the miracle of death because it would provide us with a perfect ending.

Some people, of course, might argue that nature abhors a happy death; that this fantasy goes against nature because if death were painless and worry-free, some people might prefer dying to living. I would counter that argument by explaining that life has the potential to be beautiful on its own terms, and that the vast majority of people would still choose life over death as long as they weren't suffering from a terminal disease.

Let's rephrase and qualify our fantasy. In an ideal world, how would we die? If mankind were rational and wise and mass hysteria didn't influence opinion, what mode of dying would be perfected? Let us assume that we could rise about any customs or taboos and approach death on its own terms. Let us assume that legislators, doctors, and other groups with vested interests and strong views would not attempt to impose their interests or views. All these assumptions are part of Greek philosopher Aristotle's notion of man as a primary mover, capable of selecting the primary condition of life (and death).

Given all this, that immortality is impossible and that science has made some progress in treatment of fatal diseases but that they are still with us, what would be the ideal scenario and the improvement necessary to create such a scenario?

First, we would be blessed with timely death. In other words, when organs begin to fail and life is just about to become a burden to ourselves and others, we die. Something within our bodies (or perhaps within our spirit our soul) recognizes that we are about to cease enjoying our life, perceiving beauty and appreciating what we have and pulls the plug. Certainly we could make an aspect of this fantasy real. We could set up a system where a dying person—assisted by a professional in this new science—could trigger a painless, peaceful death at exactly the right moment.

Second, the people surrounding the dying individual would support his or her decisions and not impose their own ideas or interfere with the dying process. Family members and friends wouldn't make the dying person feel guilty, ashamed, inadequate and so on. Professionals, too, would not interfere in the process unless they are part of a new breed of professionals trained in managing the dying process. This means that doctors, gerontologists and others who are trained in this process would not be allowed to make or influence the decisions many of them currently make or influence.

Continuing this idealized scenario, let's suggest five rules that might govern the process:

Rule #1: Dying patients will be approached with an open, objective mind, free from bias or pre-determined belief.

This rule means that professionals managing the care of the dying patient would be receptive to diversity. They would recognize that no two patients have the same needs; that culture, religion, socioeconomic background and many other factors determine what one person might consider an ideal death. Professionals would take a more holistic view in trying and help a patient achieve this ideal.

Rule #2: Doctors will be honest and answer truthfully all questions asked by the dying patient as well as the family.

This doesn't mean simply providing patients with the exact diagnosis and prognosis but doing so when patients are ready to hear and understand what they're told. Many times, they aren't. Doctors know that some patients aren't really listening or absorbing what they're hearing; they're in denial about their condition or they're too shocked to really understand. Other times, doctors sugar-coat diagnoses and though they tell the truth, they may not tell the whole truth or they leave patients room for hope or they don't outline all the options.

The key for this rule is that doctors need to be aware that there are certain times when patients are ready to hear the diagnosis and prognosis, and they need to read patients in order to give them information when they're able to absorb it. I've found that people are ready when they ask all the right questions. For instance, patients don't ask if they have cancer until they're ready to hear a doctor's response; they won't ask questions about the extent of the disease or the treatment possibilities until they're ready to listen to this information. An approach that I have carefully developed over the years is to inform the patient that a battery of tests (including tumor biopsy) will be done and that the results will be ready within a specified number of days, at which time I will be able to answer all questions. Those patients who are ready to hear the diagnosis/prognosis ask me the appropriate questions at the proper time, and those who are not ready, do not ask anything. I never, however, give a false diagnosis.

Rule #3: Elderly, chronically sick, and severely handicapped patients will be free to discuss their coming death.

This supposes there is a qualified person with whom to carry on these conversations. The amount of time elderly people spend ruminating about and obsessing on death is unbelievable. It is not proposed here that these deadly conversations be held with every elderly or dying patient. It is simply suggested that when the dying patient is aware that death is coming (most of the time the patient is), he should be free to discuss the coming death instead of being isolated in a hospital bed and completely cut off from the entourage. Not every dying patient likes to engage in these discussions, but many do.

Rule #4: Pharmacological drugs will be readily available to manage the conditions of terminal patients.

In other words, people would have access to whatever drug they needed in whatever quantity they required whenever they needed it. It is sad and ironic that the terminal patients for whom these drugs would be the most useful are the ones where they are used the least, especially since so much progress has been made in the development of these drugs. There is no reason whatsoever for a terminal patient to die in pain or in distress since we possess the pharmacological tools to eradicate pain and distress almost completely. Researchers, however, have little interest in dealing with terminal patients since most of the scientific research is geared toward extending life at all costs. The pharmacological activity of these drugs is well known when used in acute and chronic illnesses, but extensive statistical studies on terminal patients are limited.

Rule #5: Hospices would be used more frequently and more innovatively.

They've enjoyed some success in this country, though they're not as widespread or used as well as in England or Australia. Part of the problem in the United States is that we're so focused on prolonging life that we've neglected how to manage the end of it. Grants for protocols aimed at extending life (like a new chemotherapy protocol) are relatively easy to come by but grants for managing the end of life are relatively difficult to obtain.

In our ideal scenario, hospices will become more ubiquitous and used more effectively when:

· The dying patient is properly informed that death is coming and is properly prepared for it.

· Doctors and hospitals learn that there is a point in time when one has to stop taking care of the living and start taking care of the dying.

· The circle surrounding a dying patient stops irrationally (and often hysterically) rejecting death and starts facilitating the transition from life to death of those they care about.

· The public recognizes that there is a point when life can no longer be enjoyed and must end.

· The proper legislation makes all the above possible.

Though my ideal scenario is for people to die in the familiar surroundings of their own home, I also recognize that death at home can be frightening for family and friends. Hospices, therefore, might provide the same comfortable and familiar environment if properly managed and accepted by friends and family.

One last point about this ideal scenario: Flexibility should be built in to the management process. In other words, any approach that makes death easier is the right one, even if this approach is unconventional, antisocial or not acceptable for other reasons. To achieve a peaceful death is the goal, and that means that everyone—the healthcare professionals and family and friends—need to accommodate the wishes of the person who is dying. For many of the surrounding people this accommodation will require them to overcome their own fear of death—fear that causes them to interfere and be rigid in their beliefs. This flexibility might actually help ease the fears of those surrounding the dying patient. Too often, they witness an agonizing death and this magnifies their own fears; when they die, they are terrified because of this memory (and other similar ones). If they witness a serene, accepting death, however, they are likely to be less fearful.

Taking Responsibility for What We've Created

I would not be writing this book if it were not for the real-life scenarios humans (as opposed to nature) have produced. Only humans can function with defective organs. Our medical and technological adances have made progressive debilitation a uniquely human experience. It is the price we pay for living long and at less than 100% of our capacity.

It is up to each of us to accept that we have produced our way of dying and take responsibility for doing something about it. No one will take responsibility if they think our mode of death is fixed an immutable. While it sometimes might seem that way up close, a historical perspective reveals that it's evolving. As I've noted earlier, different societies and religions all have approached death with differences, and those societies and religions have changed their approach to death over time. Part of the evolutionary process means testing new ideas and then shaping these ideas so they work best. We need to do more of this conscious testing and shaping, since our approach to death is not going to evolve naturally or spontaneously. We have to make it.

Taking responsibility for changing our approach means that we have to extricate ourselves from the two-way miscommunication that often occurs between the dying and those surrounding them. Family, friends, and doctors are fighting to keep the patient alive because they think the patient desperately wants to stay alive. The dying patient is fighting to stay alive because he doesn't want to disappoint his doctor, family, and friends. The great irony is that everyone wants an early and peaceful death but everyone is fighting against it. The people surrounding the patient are unable to say, He wants to die; we should let him die; we should try and help the end to be as painless and as peaceful as possible. And the dying patient is unable to say, I want to die; I do not want you to interfere with my approaching death; I want you to help make my death easy.

An Optimistic View of Dying and Death

The definitive characteristic of Homo Sapiens, at least modern Homo Sapiens, is courage to change things despite fear. It is the ability to ponder on living conditions as they are, keep what is still good and then have the courage to change what is bad. The innovator may be burned alive or crucified in the process, but eventually the valuable innovation is adopted. This is how prehumans and humans looked for shelter and clothing, adopted agriculture and domesticated animals, formed societies, improved the process of human birth, split the atom, invented computers, manipulated genes, and so on. These paths are not smooth and misuse and abuse of these new innovations are always a problem. But one way or another, we manage to bring products and concepts that once were thought to be odd or worthless into the mainstream. In our own way, we're following the same crooked path with modes of dying. It's only a matter of time before we make the changes that may seem strange now but will be considered normal in the future.

Not that this process will be easy. We are burdened with an approach to dying and death that has strong, traditional roots. It takes great courage to move away from this tradition, and anyone who suggests an alternative is branded a heretic, criticized, mocked or (perhaps worst of all) ignored. There's currently a stalemate between those who want to change our approach to death and those who want to maintain that approach. I can't honestly say that we're going to move away from our irrational and unsatisfactory practices any time soon.

Still, I firmly believe that all of us are capable of changing our attitudes and behaviors in the face of death. I've seen other people—doctors, nurses, patients—change, and I know I have. People claim it is easier said than done, but I say it is easier done than said. I managed to overcome my fear and repulsion of the dying in a simple way. I remember as a young doctor when I started to inform patients of their coming deaths. Whenever I dealt with a mature and intelligent dying patient, I mentioned that I myself was scared, that I did not know how to behave and that I felt like running away. How uncomfortable I was when one day a dying patient started to comfort me: Do not be embarrassed; there is nothing to be afraid of. It is not as scary as you think. Who was treating whom? This patient and others like him dissipated my fear and antipathy toward the dying. I quickly found out that social relationships are meaningful to everyone, but they become crucial to the dying; how much more important is a positive relationship for the terminal patient than any new protocol for chemotherapy of advanced cancer?

Rationality has to replace irrationality, clear thinking has to overcome distorted emotions, logic has to obliterate obsolete customs and traditions and courage has to defeat laziness and stupidity.

I trust that all these positive attitudes and emotions will triumph in the future. The more I progress in my relationship with my patients, the more I become aware that the definition of the human condition is freedom. A human being is free when he has the ability to form an attitude or carry out a behavior that varies from the norm. The ability to change and modify a pattern of behavior handed down through custom or tradition defines our degree of freedom. An understanding and acceptance of the meaning of freedom is in the quote, I disagree with you, but I respect and defend your right to disagree with me. Reciprocally, one does not understand the meaning of freedom when one imposes one's views and does not allow others to be different. Freedom is, therefore, nothing more than respect for differences. We are not free when we choose a monotonous repetition of behavior the way animals do, when we prefer the easy pattern of an established mode when dealing with a specific situation even though it is harmful.

We need to face reality. Once we do so, we can exercise our freedom of choice. For some of us, that may mean choosing a peaceful death. For others, it may mean ending our lives weeks or even months before it's customary. For still others, it may involve seeking a euphoric death. There are many choices, and I am confident that all of us have the inner resources necessary to exercise the ones that are right for us as individuals and as a society.

There are three ways of dying:

1. The fearful way, which is more common than ever before.

2. The peaceful way, which with the recent progress in medicine and pharmacology is within reach. We can relieve physical pain and anxiety associated with death and it is the precondition for the future way of death.

3. The ecstatic way, which is very rare but could become more common since it is attainable by most of us. While some people might oppose this concept, that opposition would melt with education and prep-

aration. Greater familiarity with the Near-Death Experience could be one form of preparation to the real death experience. Montaigne said, ... in order to clear death of its misconceptions, let us deprive death of its strangeness...Let us frequent it, let us get used to it. Understanding that the beauty of life and the beauty (and serenity) of death go together and reinforce each other. We focus too much on the fear and misconceptions of death, and it is time to see the other side of it. We should talk more not less of dying and death.

Nature has not presented us with a perfect and natural way of dying. I want him to die naturally, is an impossible request because there is no natural way of dying. There are only (or mostly) man-made ways of dying.

Once we realize that we make death and usually make it the wrong way, then the next step is to make death the right way. It falls on us to make one that is suitable to our needs. In other words, the future model of death will not be a discovery, but an invention.

More research, more grants and more interest in the lives of dying people are necessary. For instance, families should have the courage to send terminal relatives to a hospice; terminal patients should also have the courage to request such a transfer. We also need to stop neglecting both the subject of death and the dying individual. If we pay more attention, we have the opportunity to make our death what we really want it to be.

The miracle of the 20th century has been the miracle of life because medical progress has solved so many of our health problems. The miracle of the 21st century hopefully will be the miracle of death, with modern pharmacology making it painless, peaceful, euphoric, and thus opening the doors for a revolutionary concept of ecstatic death.

Made in the USA
Lexington, KY
30 August 2011